REVIEW OF
Speech and Hearing Sciences

REVIEW OF

Speech and Hearing Sciences

Norman J. Lass, PhD

Professor, Department of Speech Pathology and Audiology
College of Human Resources and Education
West Virginia University
Morgantown, West Virginia

ELSEVIER

MOSBY

3251 Riverport Lane
St. Louis, Missouri 63043

REVIEW OF SPEECH AND HEARING SCIENCES

ISBN: 978-0-323-04344-1

Copyright © 2013 by Mosby, an imprint of Elsevier Inc.

Notices

Knowledge and best practice in this field are constantly changing. As new research and experience broaden our understanding, changes in research methods, professional practices, or medical treatment may become necessary.

Practitioners and researchers must always rely on their own experience and knowledge in evaluating and using any information, methods, compounds, or experiments described herein. In using such information or methods they should be mindful of their own safety and the safety of others, including parties for whom they have a professional responsibility.

With respect to any drug or pharmaceutical products identified, readers are advised to check the most current information provided (i) on procedures featured or (ii) by the manufacturer of each product to be administered, to verify the recommended dose or formula, the method and duration of administration, and contraindications. It is the responsibility of practitioners, relying on their own experience and knowledge of their patients, to make diagnoses, to determine dosages and the best treatment for each individual patient, and to take all appropriate safety precautions.

To the fullest extent of the law, neither the Publisher nor the authors, contributors, or editors, assume any liability for any injury and/or damage to persons or property as a matter of products liability, negligence or otherwise, or from any use or operation of any methods, products, instructions, or ideas contained in the material herein.

ISBN: 978-0-323-04344-1

Vice President and Publisher: Linda Duncan
Content Manager: Jolynn Gower
Publishing Services Manager: Julie Eddy
Project Manager: Jan Waters
Design Manager: Margaret Reid

Printed in United States of America

Last digit is the print number: 9 8 7 6 5 4 3 2 1

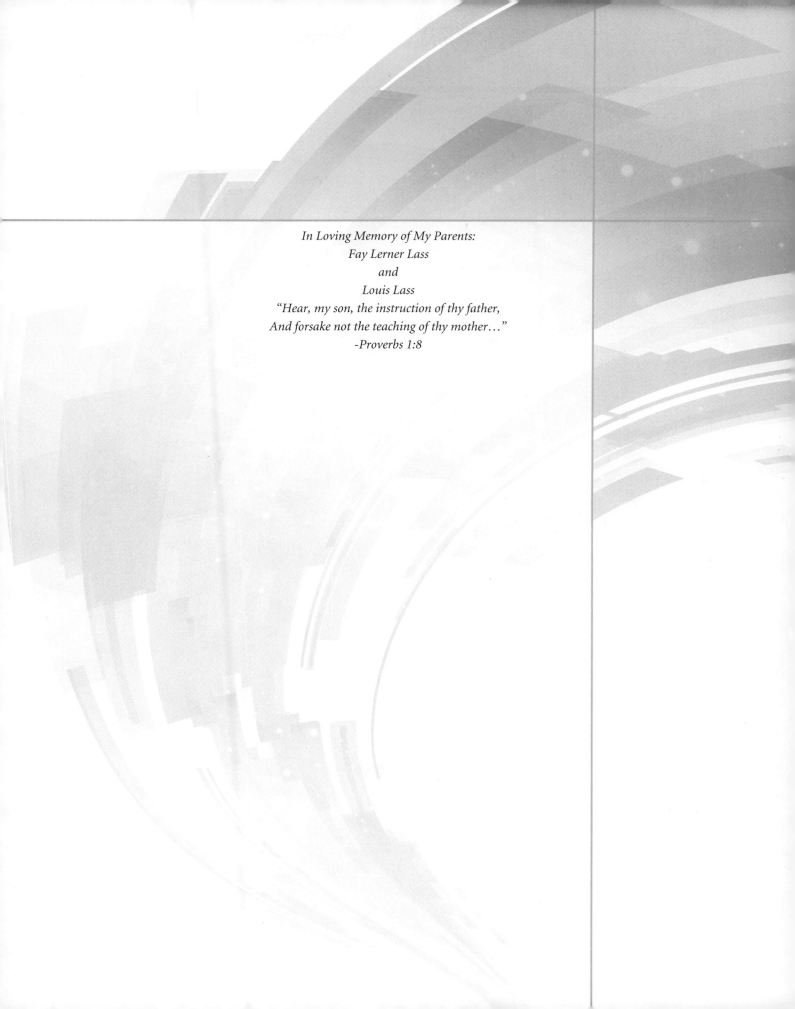

In Loving Memory of My Parents:
Fay Lerner Lass
and
Louis Lass
"Hear, my son, the instruction of thy father,
And forsake not the teaching of thy mother…"
-Proverbs 1:8

Preface

Review of Speech and Hearing Sciences is a workbook that addresses basic concepts in the speech and hearing sciences to facilitate the learning and/or review of technical material by both undergraduate and graduate students. It may be used for coursework in speech science, hearing science, anatomy and physiology of the speech and hearing mechanisms, acoustic phonetics, auditory phonetics, and physiological phonetics. In addition, it will serve the needs of students in non–science courses who would benefit from an introductory/review section of important concepts and information on anatomy/physiology as well as basic acoustics and speech acoustics. Therefore it could be used in a number of different courses throughout students' undergraduate and graduate studies. It is also intended for use in conjunction with any textbook, and therefore should be useful for all courses in the speech and hearing sciences, because it covers topics that are routinely discussed in those courses. In addition, it will be very useful as an ideal review tool for those graduate students and/or professionals who are preparing for the Praxis Examinations in Speech-Language Pathology or Audiology, because the topics included in the workbook match those that are specified in the current certification standards of the Council for Clinical Certification in Audiology and Speech-Language Pathology of the American Speech-Language-Hearing Association (ASHA).

The book contains numerous student-friendly features, including the following:

- A narrative overview in each chapter that discusses the topics of the chapter
- Anatomical and line illustrations in each chapter to help in understanding important technical concepts
- Review questions at the end of each chapter, including true-false, fill-in-the-blank, multiple-choice and, where appropriate and relevant, computational problems for review of chapter contents
- Application questions that draw on the contents of the chapter topics and their implications/applications to clinical speech-language pathology and/or audiology
- Identification questions on anatomical structures in all chapters in the Anatomy and Physiology section, with two different levels of difficulty in identifying structures of relevance to the speech production and auditory mechanisms:

Level 1 includes the names of parts of structures to identify, and the student is asked to draw a line to each part and label the part.

Level 2 includes lines pointing to different parts of each structure, but no names of parts are listed. The student is asked to identify the part to which each line is pointing.

These features make *Review of Speech and Hearing Sciences* useful not only to students in facilitating the learning/review process but also to instructors for providing a source of questions and illustrations for quizzes, examinations, and in-class learning exercises.

The book contains eight chapters divided into two major sections. The first section, **Acoustics**, contains two chapters. The *Basic Acoustics* chapter introduces students to important concepts associated with sound, including conditions necessary to create sound, properties of vibrating systems, sinusoidal (simple harmonic) motion, sine curves and their spatial as well as temporal features, and characteristics of complex sounds. Also included is a discussion of the phenomenon of resonance, specifically cavity (acoustical) resonance involving the tube model, with its analogy to the human vocal tract and the human external auditory meatus. Finally, this chapter discusses the decibel. An understanding of these basic concepts will assist readers in applying them to an understanding of the speech and hearing processes.

The *Acoustics of Speech Production* chapter addresses the acoustics associated with the speech production process. Also included in this chapter is a discussion of basic acoustic and perceptual characteristics of speech sounds, including frequency-pitch, intensity-loudness, spectrum-quality, as well as measured and perceived rate. The chapter also provides a brief discussion and illustration of the acoustical and physiological aspects of nasal sound production.

The second section of the book, **Anatomy and Physiology,** is composed of six chapters: *Respiration, Phonation, Articulation, The Conductive Auditory Mechanism, The Sensory Auditory Mechanism*, and *The Central Auditory Mechanism.*

The *Respiration* chapter describes the respiratory tract (nasal, oral, and pharyngeal cavities, larynx, trachea, and lungs), the bony skeletal framework for respiration (vertebral column, rib cage, pectoral girdle, and pelvic girdle), and the muscles involved in the respiratory process (anatomically: thoracic, neck, back, and abdominal muscles; functionally: muscles involved in the inhalation and exhalation phases of respiration).

The *Phonation* chapter addresses the larynx, a musculo-cartilaginous-membranous structure in the neck region responsible for producing all voiced speech sounds. The parts of the larynx are discussed, including the paired and unpaired cartilages of the larynx and extrinsic and intrinsic laryngeal membranes and ligaments. Also presented are the extrinsic and intrinsic laryngeal muscles and the internal cavity of the larynx.

The *Articulation* chapter contains the skeletal framework for the articulatory process, including the **cranial bones** (frontal, occipital, ethmoid, sphenoid, parietal, and temporal) and **facial bones** (mandible, maxillae, nasal, palatine, lacrimal, zygomatic, inferior nasal conchae, and vomer). Also discussed are the numerous structures involved in the articulatory process within the oral, nasal, and pharyngeal cavities, including the lips and face, tongue, palate, pharynx, and mandible.

The *Conductive Auditory Mechanism* chapter contains the structures of the outer and middle ears, including the auricle, external auditory meatus, tympanic membrane, and middle ear cavity. The detailed parts of each of these structures are illustrated, including:

- The auricle's helix, antihelix, conchae, scaphoid fossa, triangular fossa, tragus, antitragus, and lobule
- The tympanic membrane's umbo, pars tensa, pars flaccida, and cone of light
- The middle ear's tympanum and epitympanic recess, ossicular chain (malleus, incus, and stapes), muscles (tensor tympani and stapedius), as well as the fenestra vestibuli and fenestra rotunda on the medial labyrinthine wall.

The *Sensory Auditory Mechanism* chapter addresses the inner ear and its fluid-filled canals that lie medial to the middle ear cavity in the petrous portion of the temporal bone. The two separate parts of the inner ear (the bony labyrinth and the membranous labyrinth) and the structures in each part are noted along with the fluids in each labyrinth. The discussion also includes the vestibular and cochlear portions of the inner ear. The cochlea and its three fluid-filled canals (scala vestibuli, scala media, and scala tympani) are also addressed as well as the organ of Corti, with its outer and inner hair cells and nerve fibers that group together to form the cochlear nerve, and which along with the nerve fibers in the semicircular canals that form the vestibular nerve, join together to form the VIIIth cranial (statoacoustic) nerve, sending nerve impulses from the inner ear to the brainstem and eventually to the auditory cortex of the brain.

The *Central Auditory Mechanism* chapter describes the pathway of the auditory signal from the VIIIth cranial nerve to the auditory cortex. Upon leaving the cochlea, the VIIIth nerve passes through the internal auditory meatus and the auditory branch of the VIIIth nerve reaches the cochlear nucleus in the medulla, the first major nucleus that marks the beginning of the central auditory nervous system. The next major nucleus is the superior olivary complex, also in the medulla. Moving up the afferent pathway in the pons area is the nucleus of lateral lemniscus, followed by the inferior colliculus in the midbrain and the medial geniculate body in the thalamus. After this point, the afferent central auditory tract fans out into multiple small fibers called *auditory radiations*, which connect the medial geniculate body to the auditory cortex in the temporal lobe of each of the two hemispheres of the brain. The role of the auditory cortex as the primary cortical site for processing auditory information is discussed. Also addressed is the fact that the perception of loudness and pitch and other simpler auditory behaviors are controlled at the brainstem level, while higher-level behaviors (e.g., understanding speech and auditory processing of other complex signals) involve the auditory cortex's normal functioning. In addition, there is an efferent central auditory pathway of descending fibers whose primary purpose is to play an inhibitory role, preventing some afferent information from reaching higher centers.

Norman J. Lass

Acknowledgments

I acknowledge my former mentors who provided me not only with an understanding of and appreciation for the complexity of the speech and hearing mechanisms but also with the scholarly models for me to emulate. They informed and they inspired by their own scholarliness and dedication. In particular, I owe a debt of gratitude to Professors J. Douglas Noll and Kenneth W. Burk at Purdue University during my graduate studies. In addition, Professors Ralph L. Shelton and John F. Michel, faculty members at the University of Kansas during my post-doctoral studies, also served as outstanding models to emulate. The commitment of these individuals to their teaching and research has had a profound influence on my education and subsequent professional career. I will always be indebted to them.

I also acknowledge my former and current undergraduate and graduate students for providing me with the motivation to continue my teaching, research, and writing throughout my professional career. Their questions and comments have provided the basis for the contents of this volume.

I am also indebted to Jolynn Gower, Content Manager, who worked diligently and tirelessly with me on this project, as well as those involved in the early stages of this volume, including Kathy Falk (Executive Content Strategist) and Kristin Hebberd (Content Manager) at Elsevier. Their suggestions, comments, reminders, perseverance, and never-ending patience and assistance have allowed me to bring this writing project to completion. The work of Jan Waters, Project Manager, is also acknowledged. Her assistance allowed the book to be published in a timely manner. It was a pleasure to work with the staff at Elsevier because of their competence, caring, and professionalism.

I also wish to acknowledge the assistance provided by Professor Robert F. Orlikoff, department chair, colleague, and friend at West Virginia University, who critiqued the manuscript and offered very valuable comments and suggestions that have strengthened the content of the book. Finally, to my wife Martha, whose understanding and support were most helpful to me throughout the duration of this writing project my deepest gratitude and appreciation.

Norman J. Lass

Contents

Acoustics

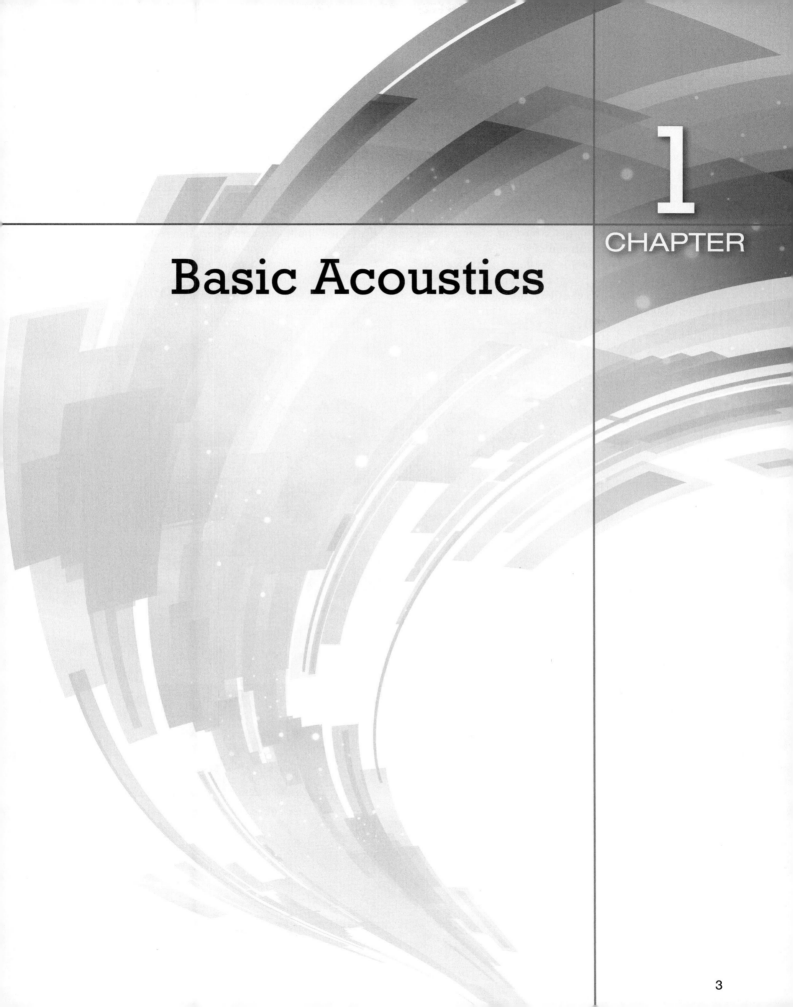

Basic Acoustics

SOUND

Sound can be defined as "a condition of disturbance of particles in a medium." Components necessary for the production of sound include: (1) an energy source, (2) a body capable of vibration, and (3) a transmitting medium. The propagating medium of most relevance for us is air. Air consists of billions of particles called **molecules**, consistently spaced with respect to one another.

The properties common to the medium of air and other media used for the transmission of sound waves are mass, elasticity, and inertia. **Mass** is any form of matter (solid, liquid, or gas). The particles in a medium, like air, consist of mass. If a medium has **elasticity**, it is able to avoid permanent displacement of its molecules. Thus it possesses the property of springiness (i.e., a propensity to return to its original position when the forces of displacement are removed). A visual aid useful for understanding these concepts is the **spring-mass model** (Figure 1-1). This model includes a mass (solid) attached via a spring to a rigid point of attachment. The mass lies on a low-friction surface and above the mass is a displacement scale. If the mass is moved from its rest position (point B) to point C on the displacement scale and is released, because of its springiness (elasticity), it will move toward its original rest position (point B). However, it will not stop there but continue moving beyond point B toward point A because of **inertia**. Then it will start to move back to its original rest position (B) because of its springiness, but again it will not stop at B but continue moving beyond B to point C, the result of inertia.

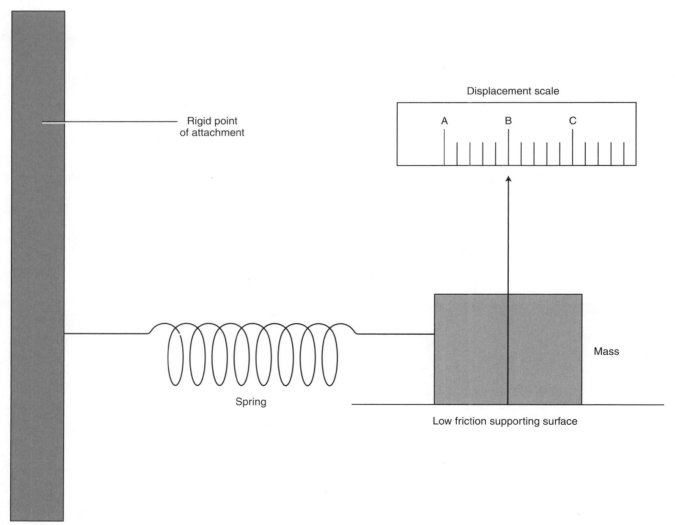

FIGURE 1-1 Spring-mass model. (From Fucci DJ, Lass NJ: *Fundamentals of Speech Science*, 1999, Allyn & Bacon, Needham Heights, MA.)

The molecules (mass) in air behave as if they had springs attached to them (springiness = elasticity), which allows them to be moved from and returned to their original rest position. However, because of inertia they do not stop. **Inertia** is a property common to all matter; it is the principle that a body in motion will remain in motion and a body at rest will remain at rest (unless acted on by an external force). Because the molecules are in motion as they move toward their original rest position, they will not stop at this position but rather will continue to move beyond it. This movement of the mass will continue until the system loses energy (**resistance**), which causes the mass to stop.

An energy source is used to activate a vibrator. Air is the energy source for speech production. However, a vibrating body will not remain in motion indefinitely because

of another basic physical property: **resistance**, which dissipates energy. The dissipation of vibratory energy is called **damping.**

Sinusoidal Motion

Because of the abstract nature of the concept of sound, visual aids can assist in describing it. One way is by discussing the simplest kind of sound wave motion that can occur in a medium. This simple wave motion is called **sinusoidal** (or **simple harmonic**) **motion.** Sinusoidal motion is a disturbance in a medium that occurs when devices such as tuning forks and clock pendulums are activated. Figure 1-2 illustrates sinusoidal motion as it is being traced from the movements of a clock pendulum.

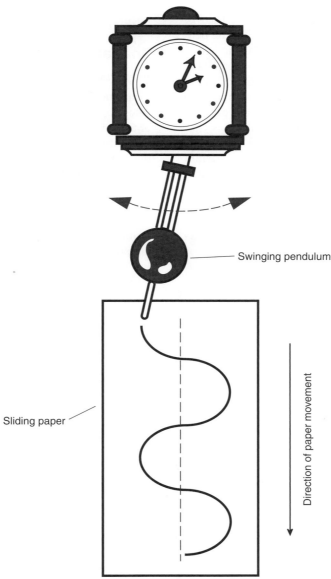

Swinging pendulum

Sliding paper

Direction of paper movement

FIGURE 1-2 Sinusoidal motion traced from the movements of a clock pendulum. (Redrawn from Fucci: *Fundamentals of Speech Science*, 1999, Allyn & Bacon, Needham Heights, MA. IN Lass: *Hearing Science Fundamentals*, 2007, Elsevier, Inc., St. Louis, MO.)

If a sheet of paper could be pulled underneath the oscillations of a swinging pendulum with a pen attached to the bottom, the picture of a sine wave would appear on the paper. The pendulum would begin its movement from a point of rest, move in one direction to a point of maximum displacement, return to its point of rest, go through its point of rest to maximum displacement in the opposite direction, and then again return to its rest position. The result is a **sine wave** tracing, which is a graph displaying two basic properties of motion: time and displacement.

The sound that is generated from vibrators that produce sinusoidal movement is called a **pure tone**, a sound that has almost all of its energy located at one frequency. However, most of the sounds that we routinely hear in our environment are complex in that their energy is concentrated at more than a single frequency.

When sinusoidal wave motion disturbs the particles of the medium, they react in a predictable way. As the pendulum or tuning fork tine begins to move from rest to maximum displacement in one direction, the particles in the medium are pushed closer toward each other; they are said to be in a state (wave) of **compression** or **condensation**. Maximum compression takes place at the point of maximum excursion of the vibrating pendulum or tuning fork tine. As the pendulum or tuning fork tine begins to move in the opposite direction, the particles attempt to return to their original positions (because of elasticity), but they overshoot that position (because of inertia) before coming to rest again. This overshoot, where the particles are spread apart more than they normally would be in their rest position, is called a state (wave) of **rarefaction** or **expansion**.

These condensations and rarefactions are the actual sound disturbances that travel through the medium from the sound source, not the particles (molecules), which simply move around their points of origin (**rest positions**). Once the sound disturbance has traveled away from the point of origin, those particles will return to their original rest positions. Thus the disturbance will have moved away from the noise source but not the individual particles in the medium; they will simply be displaced temporarily from their rest position.

The sine wave tracing can provide a spatial or a temporal picture of particle disturbances in the medium. As a spatial picture, the sine wave tracing indicates the relative positions of the particles in the medium at a single instant in time. As a temporal picture, it can be used to study the movement of a single particle over time as it changes its location around its rest position. Each view of the sine wave tracing has a set of terms associated with it.

Spatial Concepts

Amplitude

Amplitude, the maximum displacement of the particles of a medium, is related perceptually to the magnitude (loudness) of the sound. Amplitude indicates the energy (intensity) of a sound and is measured from the baseline (rest position) to the point of maximum displacement on the waveform (**peak amplitude**) or from the point of maximum displacement in one direction to the point of maximum displacement in the opposite direction (**peak-to-peak amplitude**) (Figure 1-3).

In the case of the spring-mass model, it represents maximum excursion of the mass from its rest position in one or both directions (Figure 1-1).

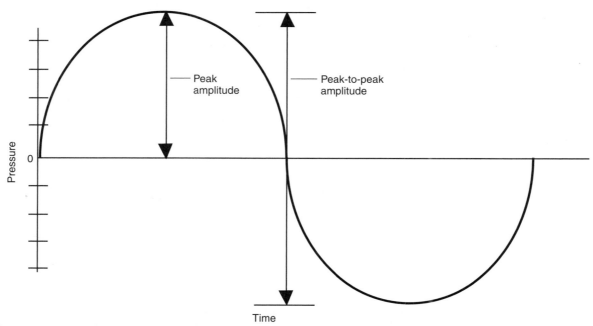

FIGURE 1-3 Peak amplitude and peak-to-peak amplitude of a sine curve. (From Fucci DJ, Lass NJ: *Fundamentals of Speech Science*, 1999, Allyn & Bacon, Needham Heights, MA.)

Wavelength

Wavelength (λ), another spatial term, is a linear measurement that refers to the distance a sound wave disturbance can travel during one complete cycle of vibration. More specifically, wavelength can be defined as the distance between points of identical phase in two adjacent cycles of a wave (Figure 1-4). (A description of phase appears in the following section.) It is inversely related to the frequency of the sound. The lower the frequency of a sound, the fewer cycles per second (cps), and therefore the longer the wavelength of the sound; the higher the frequency, the more cps, and therefore the shorter the wavelength.

Temporal Concepts

Cycle

Cycle is a time concept referring to vibratory movement from rest position to maximum displacement in one direction, back to rest position, to maximum displacement in the opposite direction, and back again to rest position (Figure 1-5).

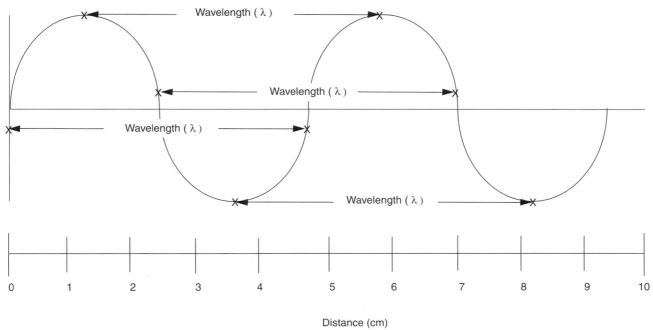

FIGURE 1-4 Wavelength (λ) of a sine curve. (From Fucci DJ, Lass NJ: *Fundamentals of Speech Science*, 1999, Allyn & Bacon, Needham Heights, MA.)

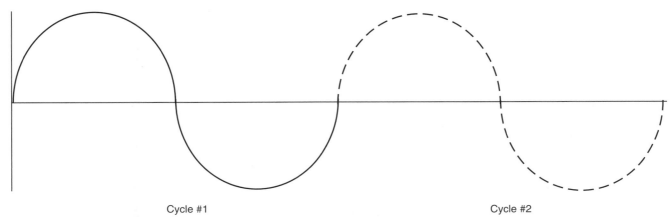

FIGURE 1-5 Cycles of a sine curve. (From Fucci DJ, Lass NJ: *Fundamentals of Speech Science*, 1999, Allyn & Bacon, Needham Heights, MA.)

Period

Period is the time (usually expressed in milliseconds) that it takes for a vibrator to complete one cycle of vibration (Figure 1-6). In the illustration the period of the sine curve is one millisecond because it took that amount of time to complete one cycle of vibration.

Frequency

Frequency is the number of complete cycles that occur during a certain period, usually 1 second. It is expressed in cps or Hertz (Hz) (in honor of Heinrich Hertz, the first person to demonstrate electromagnetic waves) or in kilohertz (kHz) (0.5 kHz = 500 Hz; 1 kHz = 1000 Hz, etc.). In Figure 1-7, the sine curve has two complete cycles of vibration in 1 millisecond, and therefore its frequency is 2000 cps, or Hz or 2 kHz (2/0.001 = 2000). That is, two

cycles in 1 millisecond (1/1000 second) results in a period of 5 msec (1 msec = 0.001 second). The **pitch** of a signal is the perceptual correlate of frequency. For example, a 100 Hz pure tone is perceived as being lower in pitch than a 1000 Hz pure tone. As was true for loudness, pitch determination is a perceptual concept and therefore requires human perceptual judgments of the sound.

Phase

Phase represents the point in the cycle at which a vibrator is located at a given instant in time. Two sinusoids are **in phase** when their wave disturbances crest and trough at the same time (Figure 1-8, *A*) and **out of phase** when they do not (Figure 1-8, *B*). Figure 1-8, *B*, shows two sine waves that are 180° out of phase.

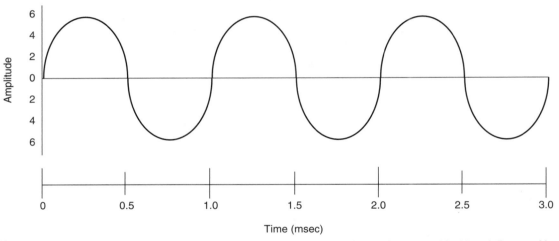

FIGURE 1-6 Period of a sine curve. (From Fucci DJ, Lass NJ: *Fundamentals of Speech Science*, 1999, Allyn & Bacon, Needham Heights, MA.)

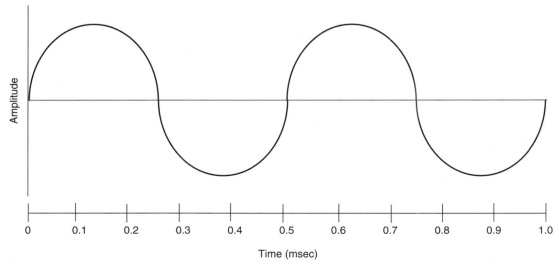

FIGURE 1-7 Frequency of a sine curve. (From Fucci DJ, Lass NJ: *Fundamentals of Speech Science*, 1999, Allyn & Bacon, Needham Heights, MA.)

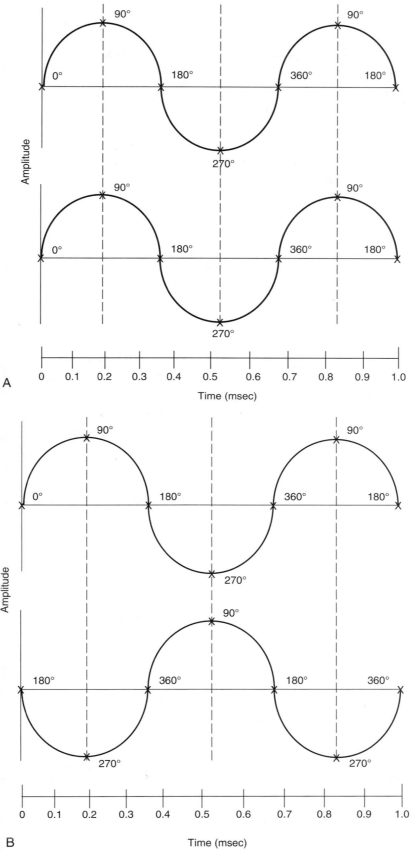

FIGURE 1-8 Sine waves in phase (A) and out of phase (B). (Redrawn from Fucci: *Fundamentals of Speech Science*, 1999, Allyn & Bacon, Needham Heights, MA. IN Lass: *Hearing Sciences Fundamentals*, 2007, Elsevier, Inc., St. Louis, MO.)

Velocity

Velocity is the speed of sound through a transmitting medium. The average speed of sound in the medium of air is approximately 1100 feet per second, or 340 meters per second, or 34,000 centimeters per second. Different sources vary slightly with regard to these figures because there are some differences in the speed of sound in air as velocity is measured at different heights above sea level and at different temperatures. The speed of sound in air is relatively constant because of the elastic and inertial properties of a given medium.

In general, the velocity of sound varies as a function of the **elasticity**, **density**, and **temperature** of the transmitting medium, with elasticity being the most important factor. The greater the elasticity of a medium, the greater the velocity; the greater the density of a medium (mass per unit of volume), the less the velocity. If we think of the particles in the two media shown in Figure 1-9 as cars on a highway, then we notice that there are many fewer cars (less mass per unit of volume, lower density) in medium A than in medium B, and therefore the potential speed of movement of cars on highway (medium) A is greater than on highway (medium) B.

Temperature has an indirect effect on velocity; an increase in temperature causes a decrease in density in a medium, which in turn causes an increase in velocity. As proof, consider this situation: if a solid is placed in an oven, as the temperature increases, the solid turns to a liquid and, eventually, to a gas. In progressing from a solid to a liquid and then to a gas via an increase in temperature, density has decreased as well (Figure 1-10).

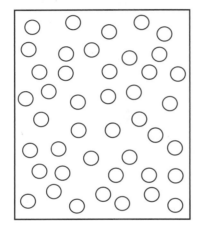
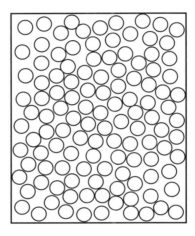

Medium A   Medium B

FIGURE 1-9 Differential density of media. (From Fucci DJ, Lass NJ: *Fundamentals of Speech Science*, 1999, Allyn & Bacon, Needham Heights, MA.)

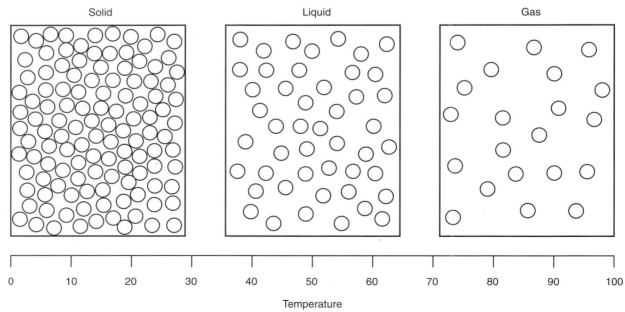

FIGURE 1-10 Effect of temperature on media density. (From Fucci DJ, Lass NJ: *Fundamentals of Speech Science*, 1999, Allyn & Bacon, Needham Heights, MA.)

Frequency-Period Relationship

There is an inverse relationship between period and frequency (Figure 1-11). This relationship is expressed in the formula:

$$Frequency = 1/Period$$

If the frequency for a particular sound wave is 500 Hz, its period is 0.002 second (period = 1/500 sec). Because period is the time needed for the completion of one cycle of vibration,

as frequency is increased (more cps), period is reduced (less time for the completion of any one particular cycle). For example, a pure tone of 100 Hz has a longer period (1/100 or 0.01 sec) than one of 1000 Hz (1/1000 or 0.001 sec).

Frequency-Wavelength Relationship

An inverse relationship exists between the time concept of frequency and the spatial concept of wavelength (Figure 1-12). As frequency is increased, wavelength becomes

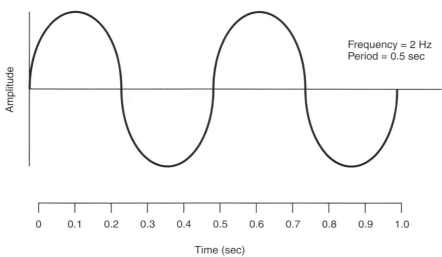

FIGURE 1-11 Inverse relationship between frequency and period. (From Fucci DJ, Lass NJ: *Fundamentals of Speech Science*, 1999, Allyn & Bacon, Needham Heights, MA.)

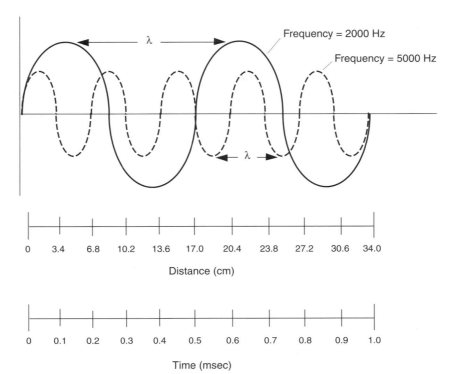

FIGURE 1-12 Inverse relationship between frequency and wavelength. (From Fucci DJ, Lass NJ: *Fundamentals of Speech Science*, 1999, Allyn & Bacon, Needham Heights, MA.)

shorter, and as frequency is decreased, wavelength gets longer. Because the number of cycles is increased within the same unit of time, each cycle takes less time and covers a shorter distance.

The relationship between frequency and wavelength can be expressed in the formulas:

$$\lambda = v/f \qquad f = v/\lambda$$

where f = frequency , λ = wavelength, and v = velocity (a constant; refers to the speed of sound).

Longitudinal versus Transverse Waves

Sound waves are **longitudinal waves**. In longitudinal waves, the particles of the medium move in the same line of propagation as the wave—in other words, in the same direction as (parallel to) the movement of the wave (Figure 1-13). On the other hand, in **transverse waves**, the particles of the medium move perpendicular (at right angles) to the movement of the wave. For example, while the wave may be moving from right to left, the particles are being displaced up and down from their rest positions (Figure 1-13). Water waves are transverse waves; while the waves are moving out in a concentric (circular) manner from the disturbance that produces them, the water particles are moving up and down, perpendicular to the wave

motion. It should be noted that although transverse waves (sine curves) are used to illustrate the various properties of sound waves (e.g., amplitude, wavelength, period, cycle, etc.), in reality sound waves are longitudinal (not transverse) waves, but their properties are more easily illustrated on transverse waves. So if we could see sound waves, they would not look like the sine curves that are used to illustrate their properties.

COMPLEX SOUNDS

So far our discussion of basic acoustics has centered around simple sounds (pure tones). When sounds of varying frequency and intensity interact, the result may be illustrated in an amplitude-by-time display called a **waveform** graph. Figure 1-14, *A* shows the interaction of two pure tones of different frequency. Another method for displaying sound is to graph it in terms of amplitude as a function of frequency. When amplitude is plotted as a function of frequency, the resulting graph is referred to as a **spectrum** (Figure 1-15).

A spectrum shows amplitude as a function of frequency at a single instant in time and has the advantage of allowing frequency to be read directly from the display. Although the spectrum provides little advantage over the waveform display when viewing pure tones (because all of the energy

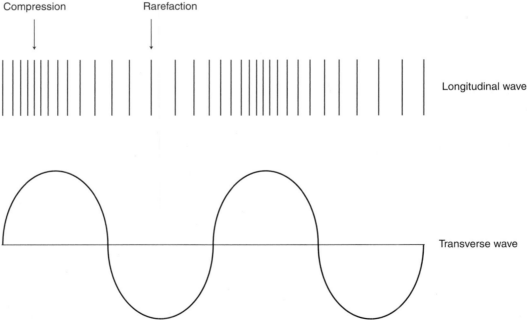

FIGURE 1-13 Longitudinal vs. transverse waves. (From Fucci DJ, Lass NJ: *Fundamentals of Speech Science*, 1999, Allyn & Bacon, Needham Heights, MA.)

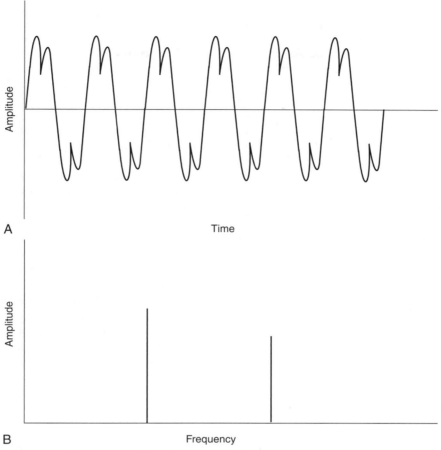

FIGURE 1-14 (A) Complex periodic waveform, (B) Line spectrum. (From Lass NJ, Woodford, CM: *Hearing Science Fundamentals*, 2007, Elsevier, Inc., St. Louis, MO.)

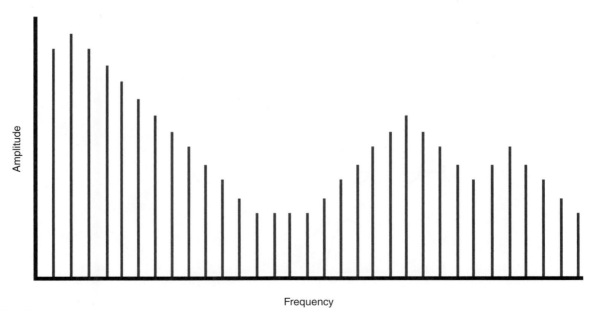

FIGURE 1-15 Spectrum of the vowel /i/. (From Fucci DJ, Lass NJ: *Fundamentals of Speech Science*, 1999, Allyn & Bacon, Needham Heights, MA.)

is concentrated at a single frequency), when viewing complex sounds in which there is energy at more than one frequency, the spectrum becomes very useful.

Complex sounds differ from simple sounds in that they have energy distributed at more than one frequency, whereas a single tuning fork generates a sound with energy concentrated at only one frequency. However, if two tuning forks of different frequencies are activated simultaneously, the sound generated consists of two frequencies and is therefore considered complex in nature. The resultant waveform no longer shows smooth curves like that of the sine wave, and the spectrum has two vertical lines, each line representing the frequency of vibration of one of the tuning forks vibrating simultaneously with the other (Figure 1-14, *B*). Speech sounds, like the vowels of English, are complex in that they have energy distributed at numerous frequencies with amplitude variations at each of the frequencies involved. Figure 1-15 shows the sound spectrum for the vowel /i/ as in b*ee*t.

Phase is the portion of a cycle through which a vibrator has passed up to a given instant in time; it is concerned with the timing relationships between individual sinusoids. Two sinusoids are in phase when their wave disturbances crest and trough at the same time (Figure 1-8, *A*) and out of phase when they do not (Figure 1-8, *B*).

Periodicity versus Aperiodicity

A periodic sound disturbance is one in which its wave shape repeats itself as a function of time and therefore has **periodicity** (Figure 1-14, *A*). A pure tone that exhibits simple harmonic motion is periodic and has a clearly defined frequency because of the periodicity of the vibrator that generates it.

J. B. Fourier, a French mathematician and physicist, discovered that any complex periodic sound wave disturbance can be mathematically broken down into its individual **pure tone** (**sinusoidal**) components of different frequency, amplitude, or phase relations with respect to one another. This mathematical analysis of complex signals into their sinusoidal components is called **Fourier analysis** (Figure 1-16). If frequency, amplitude, and phase are all considered together, Fourier analysis can be used to determine the sine waves that are combined to produce any complex periodic sound disturbance.

An **aperiodic sound disturbance** is one in which the wave shape does not repeat itself as a function of time and therefore is said to have **aperiodicity**. Static on the radio and a sudden explosion are examples of an aperiodic sound disturbance. When these sounds are heard, they are usually perceived as **noise** because they lack any cyclical or repetitive vibrations.

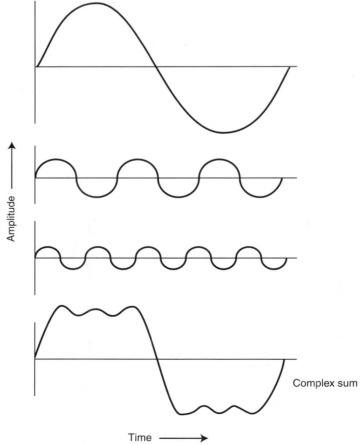

Complex sum

Time

FIGURE 1-16 Fourier analysis of a complex periodic signal into its sinusoidal components. (From Fucci DJ, Lass NJ: *Fundamentals of Speech Science*, 1999, Allyn & Bacon, Needham Heights, MA.)

Spectral displays of complex periodic and aperiodic sounds reveal the major differences between them. For complex periodic waves, the frequency of each pure tone is a whole-number multiple of the pure tone with the lowest frequency, called the **fundamental** (Figure 1-17). The first bar (i.e., the bar showing the lowest frequency) is the **fundamental frequency** and the energy bars above it, which are whole-number multiples of the fundamental frequency, are called **harmonics**. If the lowest bar of energy has a frequency of 100 Hz, then the second energy bar has a frequency of 200 Hz, the third has a frequency of 300 Hz, and so on. The heights of the energy bars for the various frequencies in this spectrum indicate the relative amplitude for each pure tone in this complex periodic sound. In this spectrum, the pure tone component with the highest concentration of energy (i.e., the greatest amplitude) is the fundamental, which is the component pure tone composing this complex signal with the lowest frequency.

For complex aperiodic sounds there is no fundamental frequency or harmonics because the disturbances produced do not display any cyclical or repetitious behavior. Instead, there is energy distributed throughout the sound spectrum at a particular instant in time. The top graph (*A*) in Figure 1-18 shows the spectrum for **white noise**, which sounds like a prolonged /ʃ/ sound. White noise has energy distributed evenly throughout the spectrum and is therefore useful for masking other sounds. Instead of having discrete lines (representing concentrations of energy or energy bars) like those used for complex periodic sound spectra, a graph or display called a **spectral envelope** is employed to indicate the distribution of energy for complex aperiodic sound disturbances, as shown in Figure 1-18, *A*.

The spectral envelope is a line running horizontally across the spectral graph, which, in this case, because it is a flat line, indicates that there is energy distributed evenly throughout the frequency range. If the spectrum is showing an aperiodic signal other than white noise, the spectral envelope would not be completely flat but would show variations where higher or lower energy regions within the frequency range are located. The lower graph (*B*) in Figure 1-18 shows the spectrum for the speech sound /s/. In this instance there is a concentration of energy in the higher frequency range and this concentration is shown by a "rise" in the spectral envelope for the frequencies where the energy concentration is located.

RESONANCE

If a periodic source of energy is used to activate an elastic system, the elastic system will vibrate at the frequency or frequencies generated by the energy source. Moreover, if the frequency or frequencies of the periodic energy source are similar or identical to those resonant frequencies of the elastic system being activated, there will be an increase in overall amplitude of vibration, a phenomenon called **resonance**. Thus resonance is the phenomenon whereby a body, which has a natural tendency to vibrate at certain frequencies (its **natural** or **resonant frequencies**), can be set into vibration by another body whose frequencies of vibration are identical or very similar to the resonant frequencies of vibration of the first body. The closer the natural frequencies of the first body to the natural frequencies of the second body, the greater the amplitude of the first body's vibrations.

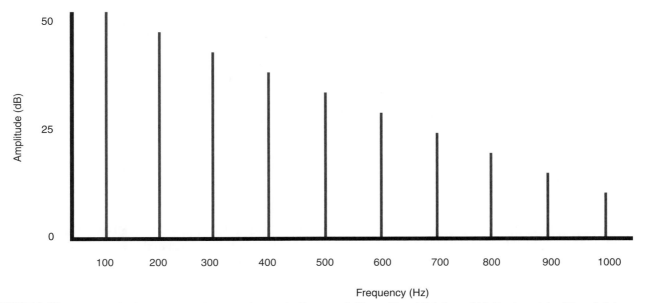

FIGURE 1-17 Discrete (line) spectrum of a complex periodic sound. (From Fucci DJ, Lass NJ: *Fundamentals of Speech Science*, 1999, Allyn & Bacon, Needham Heights, MA.)

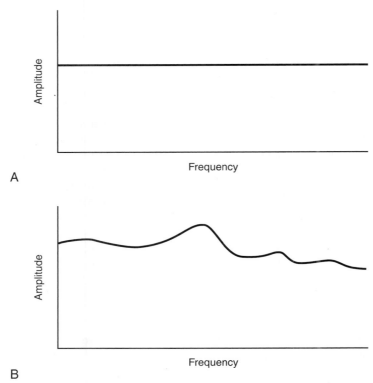

FIGURE 1-18 (A) Spectral envelope for white noise, (B) Spectral envelope for /s/. (From Fucci DJ, Lass NJ: *Fundamentals of Speech Science*, 1999, Allyn & Bacon, Needham Heights, MA.)

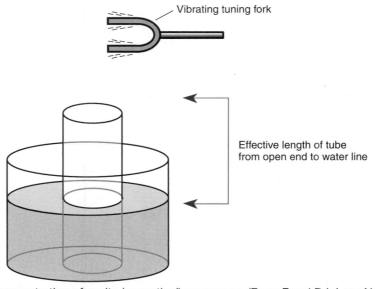

FIGURE 1-19 Laboratory demonstration of cavity (acoustical) resonance. (From Fucci DJ, Lass NJ: *Fundamentals of Speech Science*, 1999, Allyn & Bacon, Needham Heights, MA.)

Cavity (Acoustical) Resonance

The principle of resonance can be applied to the phenomenon of cavity (acoustical) resonance, a phenomenon of interest to us in understanding the speech production process. A laboratory demonstration of cavity resonance involves inserting one end of a straight tube open at both ends into a beaker of water (Figure 1-19). The open end of the tube is not submerged in the water, whereas the closed end is submerged. A vibrating tuning fork is placed over the open end of the tube, and as the tube is slowly moved up and down in the water, a certain length of tube above the water (its **effective length**) will be found that causes an increase in the perceived amplitude of the tuning fork's tone. At this point, the length of tube above the water provides the tube with the same **natural frequency** of vibration (**resonant frequency**) as that of the vibrating tuning fork. What is happening is the vibrations of the tuning fork are exciting the molecules composing the column of air inside the length of tube above the water line. Tube length is a critical factor in determining the natural (resonant) frequencies at which the column of air inside a particular tube will vibrate.

If the tuning fork in the laboratory demonstration described previously had a natural frequency of 500 Hz and was set into vibration over the open end of the tube, moving the tube up and down in the water would cause resonance to occur in the tube when its length from its open end to the water line is 17 cm (Figure 1-20). It should be noted that tube length, which has been adjusted to accommodate the excitatory frequency of the tuning fork (500 Hz), is critical to the resonance characteristics of the tube. The tube length needed for resonance to occur is equal to the λ of the frequency of the sound source (the 500 Hz tuning fork) stimulating

the tube, divided by a factor of 4, as indicated in the following equation:

$$\text{Tube length} = \frac{\lambda}{4}$$

To determine the tube length needed for resonance to occur when it is being excited by a 500 Hz tuning fork, we must first calculate the wavelength of that particular frequency. The wavelength, λ, is equal to the velocity of sound in air (approximately 340 meters or 34,000 centimeters per second) divided by the stimulus frequency, as shown in the following equation:

$$\lambda = \frac{\text{Velocity of sound in air}}{\text{Stimulus frequency}}$$

In this specific example, the wavelength for a 500 Hz signal is the velocity of sound in air divided by the stimulus frequency, which is equal to 0.68 meters (or 68 centimeters):

$$\lambda = \frac{340 \text{ m/sec or } 34,000 \text{ cm/sec}}{500 \text{ Hz}}$$
$$= 0.68 \text{ m} = 68 \text{ cm}$$

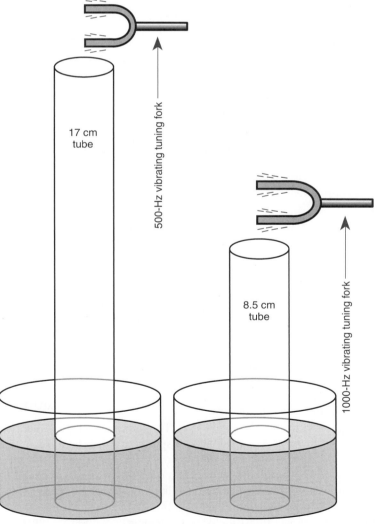

17 cm
tube

500-Hz vibrating tuning fork

8.5 cm
tube

1000-Hz vibrating tuning fork

FIGURE 1-20 Laboratory demonstration of cavity (acoustical) resonance for tubes of different lengths. (From Fucci DJ, Lass NJ: *Fundamentals of Speech Science*, 1999, Allyn & Bacon, Needham Heights, MA.)

Because the tube length needed for resonance to occur is equal to wavelength divided by a factor of 4, a wavelength of 68 cm divided by 4 is equal to a tube length of 17 cm, which is the tube length required for cavity (tube) resonance to occur when the tube is being activated by a tuning fork with a natural frequency of vibration of 500 Hz:

$$\text{Tube length} = \frac{68 \text{ cm}}{4} = 17 \text{ cm}$$

If the tuning fork had a natural frequency of vibration of 1000 Hz, the tube length needed for resonance to occur would be 8.5 cm (Figure 1-20). The wavelength would be equal to 340 meters per second (velocity of sound in air) divided by 1000 Hz (the stimulus frequency), which would be 0.34 meters or 34 centimeters:

$$\lambda = \frac{340 \text{ m/sec or } 34,000 \text{ cm/sec}}{1000 \text{ Hz}}$$
$$= 0.34 \text{ m} = 34 \text{ cm}$$

Thus the tube length needed for resonance to occur is equal to wavelength divided by a factor of 4, which is 8.5 cm when the tube is being excited by a tuning fork with a natural frequency of 1000 Hz:

$$\text{Tube length} = \frac{34 \text{ cm}}{4} = 8.5 \text{ cm}$$

Thus as the length of a tube closed at one end and open at the other end (with uniform cross-sectional dimensions throughout its length) is either increased or decreased, its resonance characteristics (i.e., its natural, resonant frequencies) are altered in an orderly pattern: as tube length is increased, the natural (resonant) frequencies of vibration for the tube become lower and, conversely, as tube length is decreased, the natural (resonant) frequencies of vibration for the tube become higher.

For example:

$$\text{Tube length} = 15 \text{ cm}$$
$$\lambda = \frac{4}{1} \times 15 = 60 \text{ cm}$$
$$f_1 = \text{Velocity/wavelength} = 34,000 \text{ cm per sec/60 cm}$$
$$f_1 = 567 \text{ Hz}$$

$$\text{Tube length} = 17 \text{ cm}$$
$$\lambda = \frac{4}{1} \times 17 = 68 \text{ cm}$$
$$f_1 = \text{Velocity/wavelength} = 34,000 \text{ cm per sec/68 cm}$$
$$f_1 = 500 \text{ Hz}$$

There is a systematic relationship between the resonant frequencies in the tube model being discussed. A straight tube (one that is uniform in cross-sectional dimensions throughout its length) closed at one end and open at the other end can be multiply resonant when excited by a sound source containing more than a single natural frequency of vibration. The first (lowest) resonant frequency for this tube of uniform cross-sectional dimensions throughout its length is equal to the frequency of a

sound wave with a wavelength four times the length of the tube:

$$f_1 = \frac{\text{Velocity}}{4 \times \text{Tube length}}$$

The tube's other (higher) resonant frequencies are odd-numbered multiples of the lowest resonant frequency. Thus its second resonant frequency is equal to the frequency of a sound wave whose wavelength is 4/3 times the length of the tube:

$$f_2 = \frac{\text{Velocity}}{4/3 \times \text{Tube length}}$$

The third resonant frequency for this tube is equal to the frequency of a sound wave whose wavelength is 4/5 times the length of the tube:

$$f_3 = \frac{\text{Velocity}}{4/5 \times \text{Tube length}}$$

For example, for a 17 cm tube, open at one end and closed at the other end, of uniform cross-sectional dimensions throughout its length (i.e., constant shape):

$$f_1 = \frac{34,000 \text{ cm/sec}}{4/1 \times 17 \text{ cm}} = \frac{34,000 \text{ cm/sec}}{68 \text{ cm}} = 500 \text{ Hz}$$

$$f_2 = \frac{34,000 \text{ cm/sec}}{4/3 \times 17 \text{ cm}} = \frac{34,000 \text{ cm/sec}}{22.67 \text{ cm}} = 1500 \text{ Hz}$$

$$f_3 = \frac{34,000 \text{ cm/sec}}{4/5 \times 17 \text{ cm}} = \frac{34,000 \text{ cm/sec}}{13.6} = 2500 \text{ Hz}$$

However, once the tube is altered so that it is not uniform in cross-sectional dimensions (i.e., a tube that is not straight), this specific relationship between the resonant frequencies no longer exists.

Thus resonance is a feature of all periodic vibrating systems that allows them to respond strongly to oscillatory disturbances that are the same as their own natural frequencies of vibration and ignoring those oscillatory disturbances at frequencies that do not match their own natural vibratory frequencies. If a system is excited at its **natural (resonant) frequencies** (those to which it most strongly responds), then it will resonate, causing an increase in overall sound pressure level (SPL).

Vocal Tract Analogy

The tube model presented previously is of interest to speech scientists because of its analogy to the human vocal tract system (Figure 1-21). The human vocal tract is composed of cavities that extend between the larynx and the lips, including the pharynx, oral cavity, nasal cavity, and the lips. Thus the human vocal tract system includes the major articulators: tongue, teeth, lips, hard palate, soft palate, and pharynx.

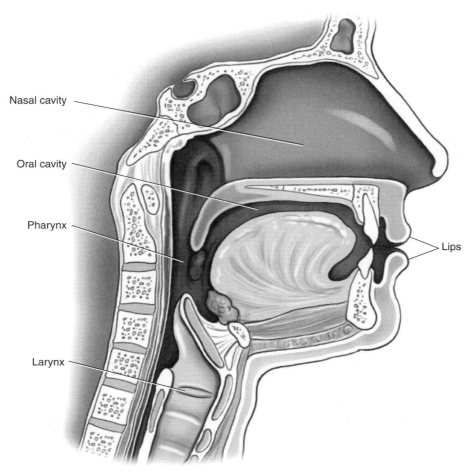

Nasal cavity

Oral cavity

Pharynx

Lips

Larynx

FIGURE 1-21 Human vocal tract. (Redrawn from Fucci DJ, Lass NJ: *Fundamentals of Speech Science*, 1999, Allyn & Bacon, Needham Heights, MA.)

The human vocal tract system is analogous to a tube closed at one end (the larynx, when the vocal folds are adducted for the production of all voiced speech sounds), open at the other end (the lips), and uniform in cross-sectional dimensions throughout its length (when producing a very low or neutral vowel sound, like /∂/) (Figure 1-22). Excitation of the vocal tract is caused by vocal fold vibrations within the larynx. The larynx produces vibrations that contain more than one frequency, and it stimulates the vocal tract from the tract's "closed end." The glottal slit between the vibrating vocal folds is so much smaller than the slit between the lips that, in a mathematical sense, the end of the vocal tract, which begins at the glottis, can be viewed as closed.

The vocal tract of the average adult male is approximately 17 cm in length when measured from the vocal folds to the lips (Figure 1-22). If this 17-cm tube is shaped for the production of the schwa vowel /∂/, it is analogous to a tube system closed at one end, open at the other end, and uniform in cross-sectional dimensions throughout its length (Figure 1-23). When excited by the complex, quasi-periodic, multifrequency sound source being generated at the larynx, this vocal tract shape allows resonances within the tube to occur at 500 Hz, 1500 Hz, and 2500 Hz. The vowel sound heard will be the schwa vowel /∂/.

The length of the vocal tract is an important factor in the phenomenon of resonance. As was the case with the tube system described previously, alteration of vocal tract length affects its natural, resonant frequencies. On average, adult males have longer vocal tracts than adult females, and adult females, in turn, have longer vocal tracts than children. Therefore vowels of adult female speakers have higher resonant frequencies than adult males and, similarly, children's vowels have higher resonant frequencies than those of adults. In each case the same vowel sound is heard, but the resonant frequencies of the respective vocal tracts are different, depending on their overall length. Therefore for every frequency there is a certain length of a resonator that will yield maximum resonance; the lower the frequency, the longer the tube or cavity.

Once the shape of the vocal tract is altered to produce any of the speech sounds of English other than the schwa vowel, the relationship between the resonances noted for the straight tube analogy no longer holds true. Thus the human vocal tract is analogous to a tube closed at one end, open at the other end, and uniform in cross-sectional dimensions, but only when it has a configuration for the neutral schwa vowel /∂/ (which is equivalent to a tube of uniform cross-sectional dimensions). However, once the vocal tract

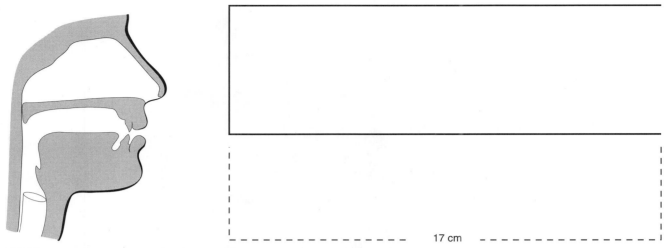

FIGURE 1-22 Inanimate tube analogy of adult male vocal tract. (From Fucci DJ, Lass NJ: *Fundamentals of Speech Science*, 1999, Allyn & Bacon, Needham Heights, MA.)

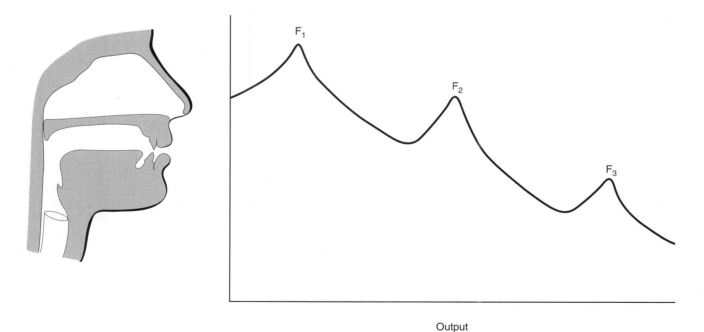

Output

FIGURE 1-23 Vocal tract output for schwa vowel. (From Fucci DJ, Lass NJ: *Fundamentals of Speech Science*, 1999, Allyn & Bacon, Needham Heights, MA.)

shape is altered to produce other vowel sounds, the analogies discussed previously must be modified (Figures 1-24 and 1-25). Thus the concept of cavity (acoustical) resonance is very important in understanding the articulatory aspects of the speech production process. The human vocal tract is analogous to a tube open at one end (the lips) and closed at the other end (vocal folds) and therefore parallels the systematic acoustic behavior associated with inanimate tubes or cavities. It is this phenomenon of resonance and its applications that relate to the acoustics of speech production.

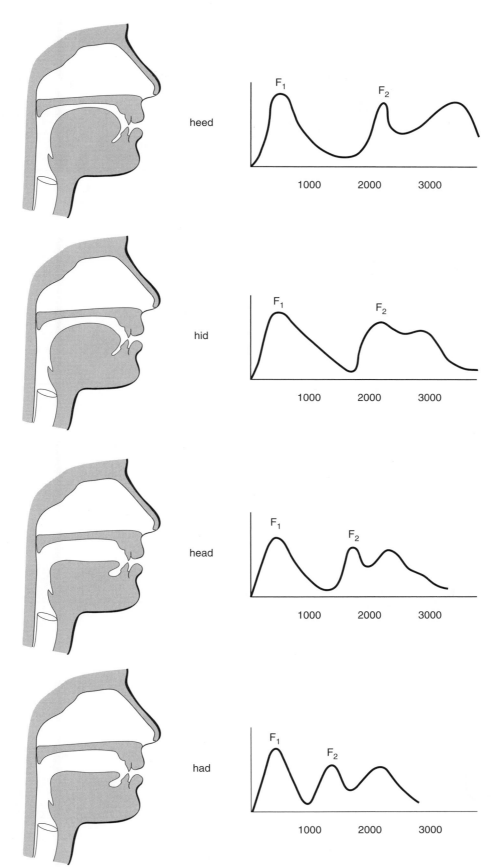

FIGURE 1-24 Vocal tract shapes and corresponding spectra for front vowels. (From Fucci DJ, Lass NJ: *Fundamentals of Speech Science*, 1999, Allyn & Bacon, Needham Heights, MA.)

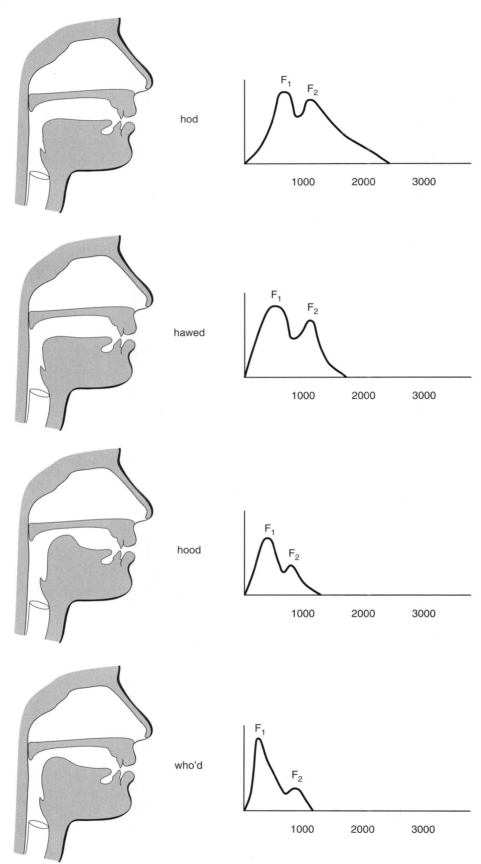

FIGURE 1-25 Vocal tract shapes and corresponding spectra for back vowels. (From Fucci DJ, Lass NJ: *Fundamentals of Speech Science*, 1999, Allyn & Bacon, Needham Heights, MA.)

Ear Canal Analogy

The tube model presented previously is of interest to hearing scientists because of its analogy to the human external auditory meatus (Figure 1-26). The human ear canal is analogous to a tube open at one end (auricle) and closed at its other end (tympanic membrane) and it is relatively uniform (but not perfectly straight) in cross-sectional dimensions throughout its length. The ear canal is approximately 2.5 cm in length from the lip of the auricle's concha to the tympanic membrane. When excited by the sounds generated by various sound sources, it responds to those sounds at its own natural (resonant) frequencies.

However, there are differences between an inanimate tube and the human ear canal. Applying the formula:

$$f_1 = \frac{34,000 \text{ cm/sec}}{4/1 \times 2.5 \text{ cm}} = 3400 \text{ Hz}$$

Research has shown that the average resonant frequency of the human external ear canal is approximately 2700 Hz. This discrepancy between the previous formula and empirical data is the result of the fact that the external auditory canal is not straight, does not have uniform dimensions,

and is not hard-walled. Thus the resonant frequency varies considerably from individual to individual. The resonance of the external ear canal provides an increase in SPL for the frequency range of 2000 to 3000 Hz at the tympanic membrane. Because these frequencies are very important for the perception of the speech signal, the concept of resonance, particularly cavity (acoustical) resonance, is very important in understanding the human auditory mechanism.

THE DECIBEL

The **decibel** (dB) is a unit of measurement to express the amplitude of an auditory signal. It is a scale based on logarithms, and is usually used to express ratios between sound pressures. The decibel is a useful means of expressing sound amplitude because of the tremendous range between the weakest sound that humans can hear and the loudest sound that they can tolerate without physical pain. The amplitude ratio of the loudest bearable sound to the faintest audible sound for human hearing is approximately 1,000,000,000,000:1 (one trillion to one), an extremely large range of numbers. The decibel scale is much more convenient because it provides a much smaller, more

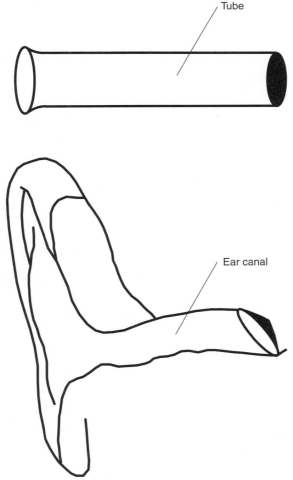

FIGURE 1-26 Inanimate tube analogy of the human ear canal. (From Lass NJ, Woodford, CM: *Hearing Science Fundamentals*, 2007, Elsevier, Inc., St. Louis, MO.)

manageable range of numbers. For example, the ratio of 1,000,000,000,000:1 can be expressed in the decibel scale as a range from **1** (the softest sound that can be heard) to **140** (the loudest sound before physical pain). Thus the decibel scale avoids the cumbersome nature of using numbers in linear, absolute scales, like power and pressure, in which all units of measurement are the same size. For example, in a linear scale of weight, the distance between 4 and 5 lbs is the same as between 50 and 51 lbs. However, this is not true of logarithmic scales, in which each unit is larger than the previous unit. In addition, unlike absolute scales of measurement that have a true zero point, the decibel scale is a relative scale in which the zero, which is used as a reference point, is arbitrary. Therefore the decibel scale expresses: (1) the ratios between two sound pressures or powers, or (2) the equivalent of a given power or pressure measurement relative to a reference point. This conversion to the smaller range of numbers is possible because of logarithms. A **logarithm** converts ratio scales into interval scales to reduce the size of the numbers required (Table 1-1).

A ratio scale is derived by multiplying the preceding number by 10 as shown in the following set of numbers: 1/1000, 1/100, 1/10, 1, 10, 100, 1000, 10,000, 100,000. An interval scale, representing the same range of numbers as the previous ratio scale, can be represented by the following set of numbers: 10^{-3}, 10^{-2}, 10^{-1}, 10^0, 10^1, 10^2, 10^3, 10^4, 10^5. The superscript number (**exponent**) in the scale indicates how many times 10 must be multiplied by itself to achieve the equivalent number in the ratio scale. For example, 10^2 (10 to the second power) indicates that $10 \times 1 = 10$, $\times 10 = 100$, which is the ratio scale equivalent of 10^2; 10 to the third power (10^3) shows that $10 \times 1 = 10$, $\times 10 = 100$, $\times 10 = 1000$, which is the ratio scale equivalent of 10^3. Thus the number 10 is the base that can be raised to some power to represent larger numbers on a ratio scale. Logarithms are the exponents to which the base is raised. The range of numbers from 1/1000 to 100,000 can be represented by the smaller set of logarithms ranging from −3 to 5, with the assumption that the base for the interval scale is 10.

The ratio between the weakest sound that can be detected and the loudest sound that can be tolerated before feeling physical pain is 100,000,000,000,000:1 (100 trillion to one). This range of sound amplitude can be represented by a factor of 14 Bels. The logarithm (to the base 10) of 100,000,000,000,000 is 14 (10 raised to the fourteenth power [10^{14}] is equal to 100,000,000,000,000 [100 trillion]). However, because the bel uses too few units (14) to represent the tremendous sound amplitude range available to human ears, the decibel (dB) (one tenth of a bel) is used. If one bel is equal to 10 decibels, then the range of human hearing can be represented by 140 dB, which is a more convenient interval scale size for expressing sound amplitudes.

The decibel can be applied to a number of scales for amplitude measurements, like the **power** or **intensity level**

TABLE 1-1   Logarithms (Exponents) to Base 10

Desired Number	Base 10	Logarithm
10	10	1
100	10×10	2
1000	$10 \times 10 \times 10$	3
10,000	$10 \times 10 \times 10 \times 10$	4
100,000	$10 \times 10 \times 10 \times 10 \times 10$	5
1,000,000	$10 \times 10 \times 10 \times 10 \times 10 \times 10$	6

(**IL**) scale, which measures amplitudes in terms of watts/cm². The lowest reference point for this scale is 10^{-16} watts/cm², which is approximately equivalent to the weakest sound amplitude that human ears can detect. The formula for expressing dB ratios when using the IL scale is:

$$\text{dB IL} = 10 \times \log R(I_1 / I_2)$$

IL is the intensity level; *10* is a constant for transforming the bel into decibels (there are 10 dB in one bel); *R* is the ratio of the intensity of one sound (I_1, the sound with the greater intensity) to the intensity of the other sound (I_2, the sound with the lesser intensity). Some examples of how this formula works are as follows:

1. If the amplitude of a sound is 100 times greater than another sound's amplitude, the dB difference between these two sounds on the SPL scale is 40 dB (dB SPL = 20 × log 100/1; 100 divided by 1 = 100. The logarithm of 100 [to the base 10] = 2; 20 × 2 = 40 dB SPL).
2. If one sound amplitude is 500 watts/cm² and another sound amplitude is 5 watts/cm², the dB difference in the IL scale for these two sounds is 20 dB IL (dB = 10 × log 500 watts per cm²/5 watts per cm² = 10; the logarithm of 100 [to the base 10] = 2; 10 × 2 = 20 dB IL).

The logarithm of a number can be obtained from log tables or a scientific calculator. In another method, the logarithm of the numbers involved could be determined by counting zeroes: The log of 1,000,000 is 6; the log of 100 is 2, and so on.

The scale most often used to measure sound amplitude is the **sound pressure level (SPL)** scale, which measures amplitudes in terms of dynes/cm² or pascals (Pa). The reference point for this scale is 0.0002 dynes/cm² (2 μPa), which is approximately equivalent to the weakest sound amplitude that humans can detect at 1000 Hz. Like the IL scale, the dB is usually used to express ratios between two amplitudes. The formula for expressing dB ratios when using the SPL scale involves multiplying the logarithm of the sound amplitude ratios by 20 (instead of 10, as was used for expressing dB ratios in ILs). The reason for this change is because intensity is equal to pressure squared ($I = P^2$). The formula for expressing dB ratios when using the SPL scale is:

$$\text{dB SPL} = 20 \times \log R(P_1/P_2)$$

SPL is the sound pressure level; *20* is a constant; *R* is a ratio of higher SPL divided by the lower SPL; P_1 is the higher sound pressure; P_2 is the lower sound pressure. Some examples of how this formula works follow:

1. If one sound amplitude is 1000 times greater than another sound amplitude, the dB difference on the SPL scale is 60 dB SPL (dB SPL = 20 × log 1000/1; 1000 divided by 1 = 1000. The logarithm of 1000 [to the base 10] = 3; 20 × 3 = 60 dB SPL).

2. If one sound amplitude is 50 dynes/cm^2 (Pa) and another sound amplitude is 5 dynes/cm^2 (Pa), the dB difference on the SPL scale is 20 dB SPL (dB SPL = 20 × log 50 dynes per cm^2 [Pa]/5 dynes per cm^2 [Pa]; 50 divided by 5 = 10; the logarithm of 10 [to the base 10] = 1; 20 × 1 = 20 dB SPL).

When they perform audiometric testing, audiologists use a measurement scale that is an offshoot of the SPL scale: the **hearing level** (**HL**; or **hearing threshold level**) scale. The zero point for this scale is elevated from the bottom of the SPL scale (0.0002 dynes/cm^2 [Pa]). It represents normal human hearing and can be different for each frequency tested because human hearing does not show the same sensitivity for each frequency. For example, at 1000 Hz, 0 dB HL is set at approximately 7.5 dB SPL. At this frequency, the average normal listener can just begin to hear a pure tone at 7.5 dB SPL. The reason for the HL scale is that some people have better than "normal" hearing (i.e., −5 or −10 dB HL at 1000 Hz). Periodically, the HL scale has been adjusted with different zero values based on more recent research findings.

REVIEW EXERCISES

TRUE-FALSE

1. Sound waves are transverse waves.

2. Sinusoidal motion is the simplest kind of sound wave motion that can occur in a medium.

3. Period is the number of complete cycles of vibration that occur in 1 second.

4. A pure tone of 1000 Hz has a shorter period than a pure tone of 250 Hz.

5. The velocity of sound through the medium of air is approximately 340 cm/sec.

6. Every cycle of sound wave vibration involves first a wave of condensation (compression) followed by a wave of rarefaction (expansion).

7. As the density in a transmitting medium increases, so does the velocity of sound waves in that medium.

8. A wave in which the particles of the medium move in the same line of propagation as the wave is a transverse wave.

9. As the frequency of a sound is increased, its wavelength becomes shorter, and as frequency is decreased, wavelength gets longer.

10. Complex periodic sounds can be mathematically broken down into their individual pure tone components that vary in terms of frequency, amplitude, and/or phase relations with respect to one another.

11. In complex periodic sounds, the frequency of each pure tone component is a whole-number multiple of the component with the lowest frequency.

12. Discrete (line) spectra are used to display the frequency and amplitude of the component pure tones that compose complex aperiodic sounds.

13. For complex aperiodic sounds, energy is distributed throughout the sound spectrum at a particular instant in time.

14. For a tube closed at one end and open at the other end (with uniform cross-sectional dimensions throughout its length), as tube length increases, the natural (resonant) frequencies of vibration for the tube become higher and, conversely, as tube length decreases, the natural (resonant) frequencies of vibration for the tube become lower.

15. A straight tube (one that is uniform in cross-sectional dimensions throughout its length) closed at one end and open at the other end can be multiply resonant when excited by a sound source containing more than a single natural frequency of vibration.

16. Cavities and tubes can serve as resonators because they contain a column of air capable of vibrating at certain frequencies (their resonant or natural frequencies).

FILL IN THE BLANK

1. The components necessary for the creation of sound include _____, _____, and _____.

2. The properties common to the medium of air and other media used for the transmission of sound waves are _____, _____, and _____.

3. The spatial concept that refers to the maximum displacement of the particles of a medium and is related perceptually to the loudness of a sound is called _____.

4. _____ is the physical property of a medium that allows it to resist permanent distortion to its original shape or its molecules.

5. _____ is the time it takes to complete one cycle of vibration.

6. The velocity of sound varies as a function of the _____, _____, and _____ of the transmitting medium.

7. _____ is a spatial concept defined as the distance between points of identical phase in two adjacent cycles of a wave.

8. A graph that displays the frequency and amplitude of the pure tone components of a complex sound is called a _____.

9. In complex periodic sounds, the pure tone component with the lowest frequency is called the _____ and the pure tone components above it that are whole-number multiples of it are called _____.

10. _____ is the phenomenon whereby a body, which has a natural tendency to vibrate at a certain frequency (its natural or resonant frequency), can be set into vibration by another body whose frequency of vibration is identical or very similar to the resonant or natural frequency of vibration of the first body.

11. _____ is a graph of the frequencies to which a resonator will respond (resonate).

MULTIPLE CHOICE

1. A physical property common to all matter that allows a body in motion to remain in motion and a body at rest to remain at rest (unless acted on by an external force) is called:
   a. elasticity
   b. impedance
   c. inertia
   d. damping
   e. none of the above

2. A time concept that refers to the movement of a vibrator from rest position to maximum displacement in one direction, back to rest position, to maximum displacement in the opposite direction, and back again to rest position is:
   a. period
   b. frequency
   c. amplitude
   d. wavelength
   e. none of the above

3. The perceptual correlate of frequency of a sound is:
   a. loudness
   b. quality
   c. pitch
   d. rate
   e. none of the above

4. Noise is an example of a _____ sound.
   a. simple periodic
   b. complex periodic
   c. simple aperiodic
   d. complex aperiodic
   e. none of the above

COMPUTATIONAL PROBLEMS

1. The period of a 50 Hz sound traveling through air is _____ sec.
   a. 50
   b. 0.02
   c. 1
   d. 45
   e. 25

2. The wavelength of a 5000 Hz sound traveling through air is _____ m/sec.
   a. 0.15
   b. 6.80
   c. 14.70
   d. 0.07
   e. 0.23

3. The frequency of a sound wave traveling through the medium of air with a wavelength of 60 cm is _____ Hz.
   a. 566.67
   b. 0.05
   c. 0.18
   d. 18.83
   e. 5.67

4. If the fundamental of a complex periodic sound is 500 Hz, the eighth harmonic of this sound is _____ Hz.
   a. 8000
   b. 4000
   c. 1300
   d. 40,000
   e. 1000

5. For an inanimate tube closed at one end and open at the other end, of uniform cross-sectional dimensions throughout its length, the third resonant frequency is equal to the frequency of a sound wave whose wavelength is _____ times the length of the tube.
   a. 4
   b. 4/3
   c. 3
   d. 4/5
   e. 1

6. The tenth resonant frequency of a 20-m tube closed at one end and open at the other end of uniform cross-sectional dimensions throughout its length is _____ Hz.
   a. 4.2
   b. 81

c. 8095.2
d. 261.9
e. 34

7. The pressure of sound X is 10,000 dynes /cm^2 (Pa) and the pressure of sound Y is 100 dynes /cm^2 (Pa). How many dB greater is sound X than sound Y?
   a. 20 dB
   b. 10 dB
   c. 40 dB
   d. 100 dB
   e. none of the above

8. The power of sound A is 5000 watt/cm^2 and the power of sound B is 5,000,000 watt/cm^2. How many dB greater is sound B than sound A?
   a. 40 dB
   b. 100 dB
   c. 60 dB
   d. 20 dB
   e. none of the above

9. The pressure of sound Z is 75 dynes /cm^2 (Pa). What is its intensity in dB?

   a. $10 \times \log \dfrac{75 \text{ dynes/cm}^2(\text{Pa})}{0.0002 \text{ dynes/cm}^2(\text{Pa})}$

   b. $20 \times \log \dfrac{75 \text{ dynes/cm}^2(\text{Pa})}{10^{-16} \text{ dynes/cm}^2(\text{Pa})}$

   c. $20 \times \log \dfrac{75 \text{ dynes/cm}^2(\text{Pa})}{0.0002 \text{ dynes/cm}^2(\text{Pa})}$

   d. $10 \times \log \dfrac{75 \text{ dynes/cm}^2(\text{Pa})}{10^{-16} \text{ dynes/cm}^2(\text{Pa})}$

   e. none of the above

10. The power of sound Z is 2000 watt/cm^2. What is its intensity in dB?

    a. $10 \times \log \dfrac{2000 \text{ watt/cm}^2}{0.0002 \text{ watt/cm}^2}$

    b. $20 \times \log \dfrac{2000 \text{ watt/cm}^2}{10^{-16} \text{ watt/cm}^2}$

    c. $20 \times \log \dfrac{2000 \text{ watt/cm}^2}{0.0002 \text{ watt/cm}^2}$

    d. $10 \times \log \dfrac{2000 \text{ watt/cm}^2}{10^{-16} \text{ watt/cm}^2}$

    e. none of the above

Acoustics of Speech Production

Speech production is a very complicated process. However, the acoustics of speech production provide an opportunity to view this complex process in a simpler manner and thus to make inferences about the speech production process.

ACOUSTICAL MODEL OF SPEECH PRODUCTION

The **acoustic theory of vowel production** (also called the **source-filter theory**) resulted from the study of the acoustical signal that is generated during the speech production process. This theory was proposed by Dr. Gunnar Fant of the Royal Transmission Laboratory in Stockholm, Sweden, in his publication, *Acoustic Theory of Speech Production*. It explains how sound produced at the level of the larynx is modified by the filtering system of the vocal tract as a result of altering vocal tract resonances, thereby allowing us to produce different vowels. The theory contains the three elements involved in vowel production: the glottal sound, the vocal tract resonator, and the sound at the lips (Figure 2-1).

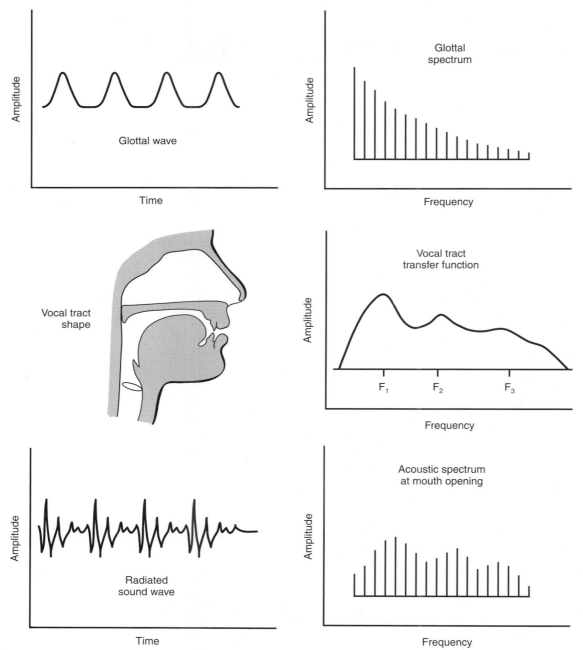

FIGURE 2-1 Three elements of the source-filter theory involved in vowel production. (Adapted from Fant G: *Acoustic Theory of Speech Production,* 1960, Mouton, The Hague.)

The glottal sound, the sound at the level of the larynx, is represented by the glottal spectrum in Figure 2-1. The fundamental frequency (f_0), the pure tone component of the complex quasiperiodic signal of the vocal folds with the lowest frequency, has the greatest amplitude with a 12-decibel (dB) octave drop in amplitude for the higher pure tone components above the fundamental.

The parts of the body involved in speech production include the lungs, trachea, larynx, pharynx, nasal cavity, and oral cavity, forming a tube that extends from the lungs to the lips (Figure 2-2). The part of this tube that extends from the glottis to the lips is called the **vocal tract**, and consists of the pharynx, oral cavity, and nasal cavity (Figure 2-3). Its shape can be varied extensively by movements of the articulators.

The conditions necessary for the production of sound waves are a source of energy, vibrator, and transmitting medium. For speech production, the source of energy is the steady stream of air that comes from the lungs when we exhale. Although this airstream is inaudible during normal breathing, it can be made audible by setting it into vibration, and this is what happens during the speech production process by means of a vibratory mechanism.

Vocal Folds

There are several ways to set this airstream into vibration; the most common method is that of vocal fold vibration. The two vocal folds are part of the larynx and provide an adjustable barrier across the airstream coming from the lungs.

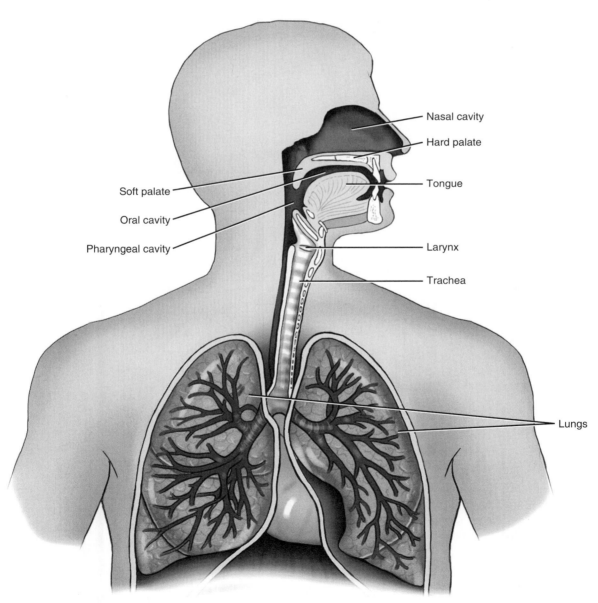

FIGURE 2-2 Parts of the body forming a tube involved in speech production.

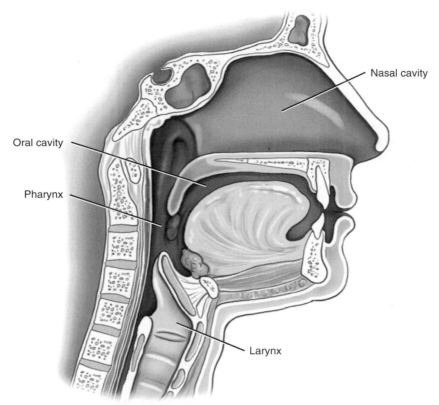

FIGURE 2-3 Vocal tract, the portion of the tube extending from the glottis to the lips. (Redrawn from Fucci DJ, Lass NJ: *Fundamentals of Speech Science*, 1999, Allyn & Bacon, Needham Heights, MA.)

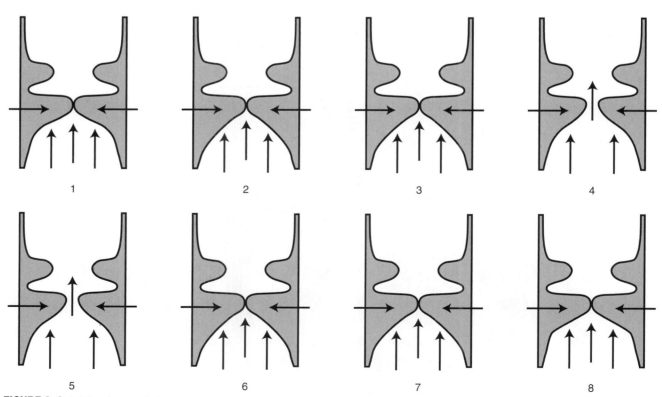

FIGURE 2-4 Adduction and abduction of the vocal folds. (From Fucci DJ, Lass NJ: *Fundamentals of Speech Science*, 1999, Allyn & Bacon, Needham Heights, MA.)

When they are open (**abduction**), the airstream passes into the vocal tract with no interference. However, when they are closed (**adduction**), they block the airstream and thus shut off air flow from the lungs (Figure 2-4).

When the vocal folds approximate in midline, subglottic pressure is built up beneath them. If this pressure is great enough, the folds are forced apart and the air in the lungs is released. The opening-closing motion of the folds gives rise to a **complex**, **quasiperiodic signal** with a spectrum of a large number of component frequencies that are whole-number multiples of the lowest frequency (which is called the **fundamental frequency** of the voice and is directly determined by the frequency of the vocal folds' vibrations).

When voiced speech sounds are produced, the vocal folds open and close rapidly, chopping up the steady airstream into a series of puffs and thus producing a buzz-like sound. The puffs of air emitted from the folds then move up through the vocal tract (pharynx, oral cavity, and nasal cavity) and out the lips (or nostrils). The vocal tract has an effect on this buzzlike sound. The shape of the vocal tract affects its acoustic properties, which in turn affect the character of the buzzlike sound that is emitted from the vocal folds (Figure 2-1).

Physiologically, during speech, the shape of the vocal tract is continually altered by articulatory movements, and it is these movements that by altering the acoustic properties of the vocal tract enable the production of different speech sounds. Therefore the steady air flow from the lungs provides the energy for speech production, and the vocal folds serve as the vibrator, converting this energy into an audible buzz. Then the articulators alter the shape of the vocal tract, which converts this buzz into distinguishable speech sounds. Thus articulation is accomplished by adjusting the vocal tract's shape to produce different speech sounds. This mechanism is responsible for producing all voiced speech sounds, which include all vowels, diphthongs, and voiced consonants.

Another method for making the airstream from the lungs audible involves constriction of the vocal tract at some point along its length, and the airstream passing through the constriction becomes turbulent. This turbulent airstream produces the hissing sound of fricatives: /s/, /ʃ/, /z/, /ð/, /ʒ/, /f/, and /v/. Still another method for producing speech sounds is to stop the flow of air completely, but only momentarily, by blocking the vocal tract with the tongue or lips, and then suddenly releasing the air pressure built up behind this air blockage. This method is used to produce the plosive consonants /p/, /b/, /t/, /d/, /k/, and /g/. It should be noted that these two methods are independent of vocal fold activity, thus allowing for the simultaneous vibration of the vocal folds for voiced consonants and no vocal fold activity for voiceless consonants. Therefore a combination of the two mechanisms is possible, as in: /b/, /d/, /g/, /z/, /ð/, /v/, and /dʒ/ (i.e., voiced plosive, fricative, and affricate sounds).

Vocal Tract

The vocal tract is an air-filled tube and, like all air-filled tubes, can act as a resonator. This means that the vocal tract has certain natural (resonant) frequencies of vibration, and that it responds more readily to sound waves with frequencies the same as its own natural resonant frequencies than to sound waves of other frequencies. Thus when the quasiperiodic wave produced at the vocal folds is transmitted through the vocal tract, the tract will respond better to those components of the vocal fold puffs that are at or near its **natural (resonant) frequencies**. These components are emphasized and the spectrum of the sound emerging from the lips will exhibit a peak at each of the natural frequencies of the vocal tract. The **transfer function** is the frequency response curve of the human vocal tract. (Figures 2-1 and 2-5)

Therefore the pulses that are emitted from the folds provide a sharp tap on the air in the vocal tract, and this air is set into vibration. However, it should be noted that the

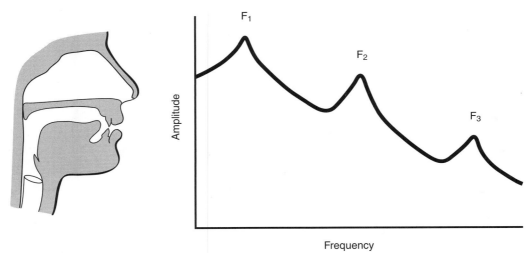

FIGURE 2-5 Vocal tract shape and resultant spectral envelope. (From Fucci DJ, Lass NJ: *Fundamentals of Speech Science*, 1999, Allyn & Bacon, Needham Heights, MA.)

movements of the vocal folds are not sufficient by themselves to set up vibrations that are heard as sounds. This requires the action of the vocal tract, which acts as a resonator (i.e., it will respond differentially to components of the complex quasiperiodic pulses that are generated by the

vocal folds). Moreover, because the vocal tract is a multiply resonant tube, it emphasizes harmonics of the vocal fold pulses at a number of different frequencies. The spectrum of the speech wave has a peak for each of the vocal tract's natural (resonant) frequencies (Figure 2-6).

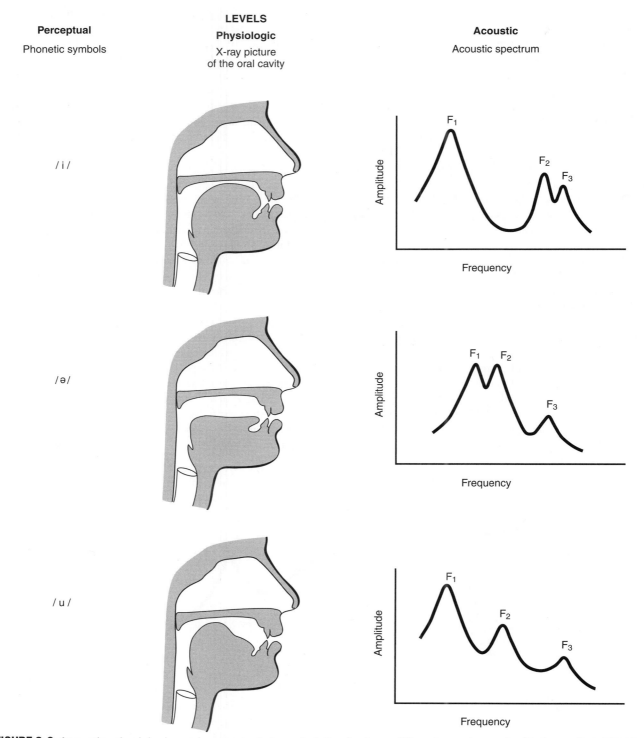

FIGURE 2-6 Acoustic, physiologic, and perceptual characteristics for three different vowel sounds. (Redrawn from Fucci DJ, Lass NJ: *Fundamentals of Speech Science*, 1999, Allyn & Bacon, Needham Heights, MA.)

The resonances of the vocal tract are called **formants**, and the frequencies of these formants are called **formant frequencies**. The quantitative values of the formant frequencies are determined by the shape of the vocal tract, which in turn is largely determined by articulatory movements in the tract. Thus every different configuration of the vocal tract has its own unique set of characteristic formant frequencies (Figure 2-6).

Because each vowel sound requires a different configuration (shape) of the vocal tract (which is accomplished by movement of the articulators), and each configuration of the vocal tract has its own characteristic formant frequencies, then each vowel sound, which represents a distinct configuration of the vocal tract, has its own unique set of characteristic formant frequencies, as evidenced by the differences in the speech spectra of the different vowels. The formants of each vowel sound are largely responsible for the characteristic quality of each vowel (e.g., /i/ vs. /u/ vs. /∂/, etc.) (Figure 2-7).

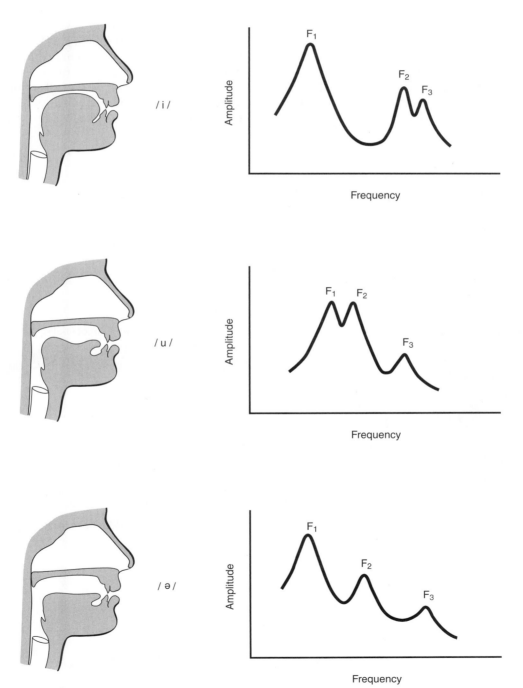

FIGURE 2-7 Relationship of vocal tract shapes and spectral envelopes for three different vowels. (Redrawn from Fucci DJ, Lass NJ: *Fundamentals of Speech Science*, 1999, Allyn & Bacon, Needham Heights, MA.)

The peaks in the spectra of vowels, the regions in which the frequency components are relatively high in amplitude, correspond to the formants (the resonant frequencies of the air in the vocal tract). Thus the formant frequencies of each vowel differ from every other vowel's formant frequencies because the shape of the vocal tract differs for each vowel (Figure 2-7).

The quantitative values of vowels' formant frequencies depend on three physiological factors:

1. The size (or cross-sectional area or radius) of the maximum constriction (which is controlled by tongue movement relative to its distance from the roof of the mouth)
2. The position of the point of maximum constriction in the vocal tract (which is controlled by tongue movement relative to its distance from the glottis)
3. The position of the lips (liprounding) (Figure 2-8)

The specific physical rules to determine the quantitative differences in formants based on the configuration of the vocal tract, a multiply-resonant tube (resonator), are discussed in the following paragraphs.

Rules for First Formant

For front vowels, the chief cause of variation in the first formant (F_1) is variation in the size (or cross-sectional area or radius) of the maximum constriction in the vocal tract, which is determined by the height of the tongue in the oral cavity. It is the space between the tongue and the roof of the mouth. The rule states that as the cross-sectional area (radius, size) of the maximum constriction of the vocal tract increases, F_1 also increases. Thus high front vowels have the lowest F_1 and low front vowels have the highest F_1.

For back vowels, variation in F_1 is largely determined by the position of the point of maximum constriction relative to its distance from the glottis. The rule states that as the point of maximum constriction moves farther from the glottis, F_1 decreases. Thus high back vowels have the lowest F_1 and low back vowels have the highest F_1 (Figures 2-9 and 2-10).

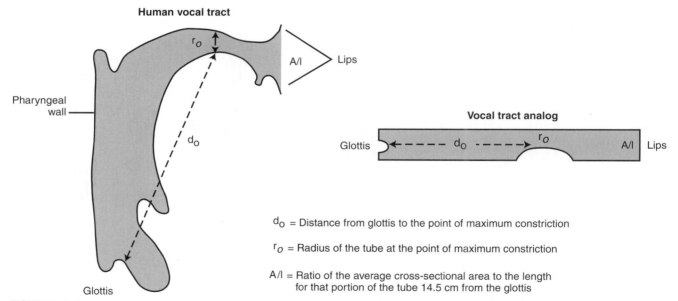

FIGURE 2-8 Three physiological factors that determine the quantitative values of vowels' formant frequencies. (Adapted from Fant G: *Acoustic Theory of Speech Production*, 1960, Mouton, The Hague.)

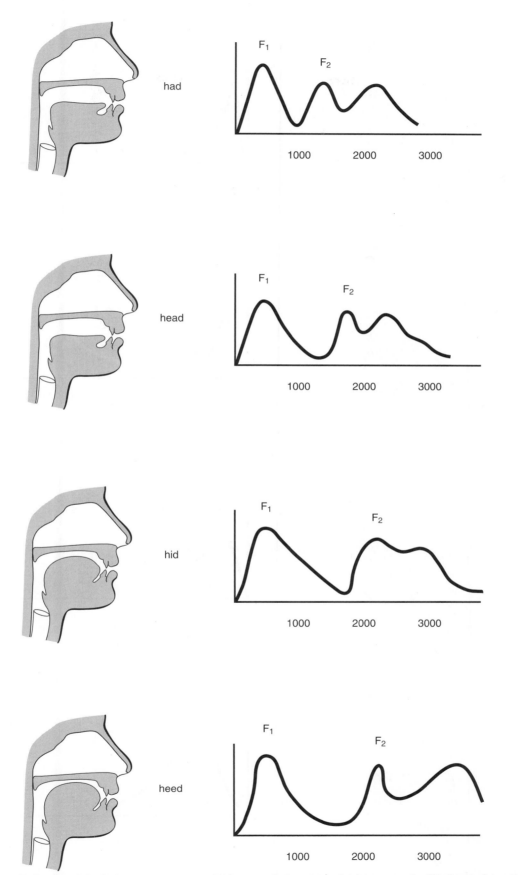

FIGURE 2-9 Variations in vocal tract shape and resultant formant frequencies for front vowels. (Redrawn from Fucci DJ, Lass NJ: *Fundamentals of Speech Science*, 1999, Allyn & Bacon, Needham Heights, MA.)

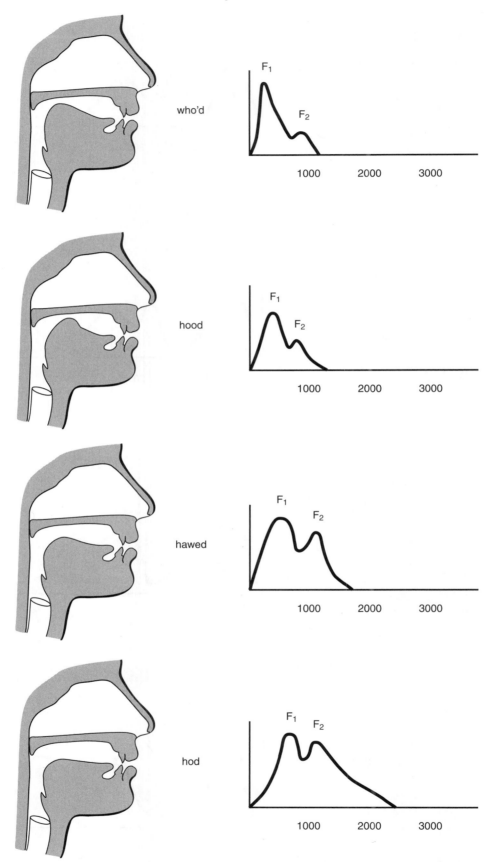

FIGURE 2-10 Variations in vocal tract shape and resultant formant frequencies for back vowels. (Redrawn from Fucci DJ, Lass NJ: *Fundamentals of Speech Science*, 1999, Allyn & Bacon, Needham Heights, MA.)

Rules for Second Formant

For front vowels, the chief cause of variation in the second formant (F_2) is the same as for F_1: variation in the size (or cross-sectional area or radius) of the maximum constriction in the vocal tract. However, the rule is reversed for F_2. It states that as the cross-sectional area (radius, size) of the maximum constriction of the vocal tract increases, F_2 decreases. Thus high front vowels have the highest F_2 and low front vowels have the lowest F_2 (Figures 2-9 and 2-10).

For back vowels, a major factor responsible for variations in F_2 is liprounding, which causes a decrease in frequency (as well as amplitude) of F_2. In fact, it is lip movement rather than tongue movement that is responsible for the lowering of F_2.

It should be noted here that voiced consonants also depend on the pulses from the vocal folds for setting the air in the vocal tract into vibration. For each consonant sound (just as there was for each vowel sound), there are characteristic positions of the articulators and therefore a characteristic set of formant frequencies.

Thus there are two systems operating in the speech production process: (1) a **generator system** responsible for producing the fundamental frequency and harmonics of the voice and (2) a **resonator system** that determines the formant frequencies of the vocal tract. These two distinct systems operate independently of each other, and therefore it is possible to alter the fundamental frequency of the voice without changing the formant frequencies of speech sounds, as well as to change the formant frequencies of speech sounds without also altering the vocal fundamental frequency.

For example, the vowel /ə/ can be produced using different vocal pitches (Figure 2-11). The formant frequencies (resonator system) for /ə/ remain approximately the same (approximately the same vocal tract configuration is used), but the vocal fundamental frequency and harmonics (generator system) vary for the various pitches used. Conversely, we can produce the vowels /u/, /i/, and /a/ at approximately the same pitch (Figure 2-7), which will alter the formant frequencies of the resonator system (because of the different vocal tract configurations required for the three different vowels), but with approximately the same vocal fundamental frequency and harmonics of the generator system.

Moreover, in general, the frequencies of the formants are not necessarily the same as those of the harmonics, because each is determined by a different system and the two systems function independently of each other. It should be noted that the vocal tract does not affect the frequency of the fundamental and harmonics; it simply emphasizes (resonates) those harmonics that happen to be similar to its own natural, resonant frequencies.

Quantitative Determination of the Vocal Tract's Formant Frequencies

Although it has been determined that the formant frequencies of the vocal tract differ for each vowel because the configuration of the vocal tract differs for the production of each vowel, the question remains as to how the different quantitative values of the formant frequencies of the different vowels are determined. The answer lies in the discussion of the phenomenon of resonance in tubes as discussed in Chapter 1. Air-filled tubes can act as resonators, and the air in a tube follows physical laws for determining the resonant frequencies of tubes. Because of its analogy to the human speech production mechanism, the laws employed for the determination of resonant frequencies of a tube closed at one end and open at the other end are applicable to the human vocal tract (Figure 2-12). The vocal tract is considered to be a tube open at one end (the lips) and closed at the other end (the glottis, when the vocal folds are approximated), approximately 17 cm (for adult males) (and approximately 15 cm for adult females) in length (L). Therefore the rules for calculation of resonant frequencies in inanimate tubes open at one end and closed at the other end are applicable for the calculation of resonant (formant) frequencies of the human vocal tract.

The physical rules are as follows:

1. The lowest resonant (formant) frequency is equal to the frequency of a sound wave with a wavelength (λ) four times the length of the tube.
2. The value of the tube's other higher resonant (formant) frequencies have wavelengths that are odd-numbered multiples ($4/2n - 1 \times L$) of this lowest resonant (formant) frequency.

$$F_n = \frac{v}{\lambda_n}$$

$$F_1 = \frac{v}{4/1 \times L} \quad F_2 = \frac{v}{4/3 \times L} \quad F_3 = \frac{v}{4/5 \times L} \quad F_4 = \frac{v}{4/7 \times L} \text{ etc.}$$

The first (lowest) resonant frequency for this tube of uniform cross-sectional dimensions throughout its length is equal to the frequency of a sound wave with a wavelength (λ) four times the length of the tube:

$$F_1 = \frac{\text{Velocity}}{4/1 \times \text{Tube length}}$$

The tube's other (higher) resonant frequencies have wavelengths that are odd-numbered multiples of the lowest resonant frequency. Thus its second resonant frequency is equal to the frequency of a sound wave with a wavelength 4/3 times the length of the tube:

$$F_2 = \frac{\text{Velocity}}{4/3 \times \text{Tube length}}$$

The third resonant frequency for this tube is equal to the frequency of a sound wave with a wavelength 4/5 times the length of the tube:

$$F_3 = \frac{\text{Velocity}}{4/5 \times \text{Tube length}}$$

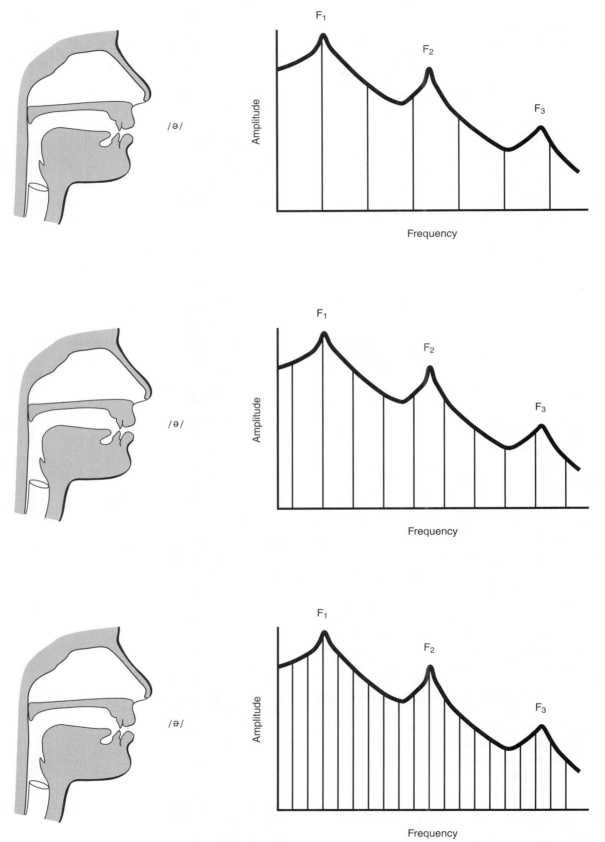

FIGURE 2-11 Illustration of the independence of the generator and resonator systems in speech production. (Redrawn from Fucci DJ, Lass NJ: *Fundamentals of Speech Science*, 1999, Allyn & Bacon, Needham Heights, MA.)

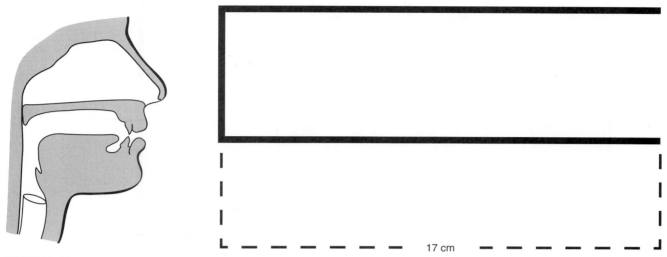

FIGURE 2-12 Analogy of an inanimate tube closed at one end to the human vocal tract and its resonant properties. (From Fucci DJ, Lass NJ: *Fundamentals of Speech Science*, 1999, Allyn & Bacon, Needham Heights, MA.)

And so on. For example, for a 17-cm tube open at one end and closed at the other end and of uniform cross-sectional dimensions throughout its length (i.e., constant shape):

$$F_1 = \frac{34{,}000 \text{ cm/sec}}{4/1 \times 17 \text{ cm}} = \frac{34{,}000 \text{ cm/sec}}{68 \text{ cm}} = 500 \text{ Hz}$$

$$F_2 = \frac{34{,}000 \text{ cm/sec}}{4/3 \times 17 \text{ cm}} = \frac{34{,}000 \text{ cm/sec}}{22.67 \text{ cm}} = 1500 \text{ Hz}$$

$$F_3 = \frac{34{,}000 \text{ cm/sec}}{4/5 \times 17 \text{ cm}} = \frac{34{,}000 \text{ cm/sec}}{13.6 \text{ cm}} = 2500 \text{ Hz}$$

Thus we can calculate any of the formant frequencies of the vocal tract. However, although the tract is a multiply resonant tube, usually we are concerned only with the first two or three formants because they are adequate for recognition and distinction of one vowel from another.

The adult male vocal tract is approximately 17 cm in length from the glottis to the lips. For this tube, provided it has a uniform cross-sectional area along its entire length (the same shape and size), the principal formant frequencies are approximately the following:

$F_1 = 500$ Hertz (Hz)
$F_2 = 1500$ Hz
$F_3 = 2500$ Hz

The adult female vocal tract is approximately 15 cm in length from the glottis to the lips. For this tube, provided it has a uniform cross-sectional area along its entire length (the same shape and size), the principal formant frequencies are approximately the following:

$F_1 = 567$ Hz
$F_2 = 1700$ Hz
$F_3 = 3400$ Hz

However, the human vocal tract is a complex resonator, constantly changing its shape for the production of different speech sounds. Consequently, its formant frequencies are not as regularly spaced as for a uniform tube. It is a nonuniform tube. In other words, its cross-sectional area varies considerably along its length, and to the degree to which its cross-sectional area is not uniform, its formant frequencies are different from those based on the acoustic theory's inanimate tube model of the vocal tract. This is a very important concept in helping us understand the speech production process and the acoustics of speech.

By means of analysis of the spectra of vowels of American English, we have been able to establish the actual formant frequencies of these vowels produced by human speakers. It has been discovered that there is considerable variability in the frequencies of formants of different vowels. Moreover, the range of formant frequencies produced when any one vowel is uttered overlaps the range of adjacent vowels, a not surprising finding in that the corresponding articulatory configurations to produce the different vowels are equally variable and overlapping. The production of vowels is variable and sometimes similar to the configurations used for the production of contiguous vowels (e.g., /i/ and /I/, /u/ and /ʊ/, etc.).

Nasal Sound Production

For nasal consonants the **soft palate** (**velum**) is lowered, thus coupling the nasal and oral cavities. The result of this coupling is basically a different vocal tract shape. The vocal tract starts as a single tube in the pharynx but separates into two branches at the soft palate, with one branch going through the nasal cavity and the other going through the oral cavity. The result of this different vocal tract configuration is a different set of formant frequencies (Figure 2-13).

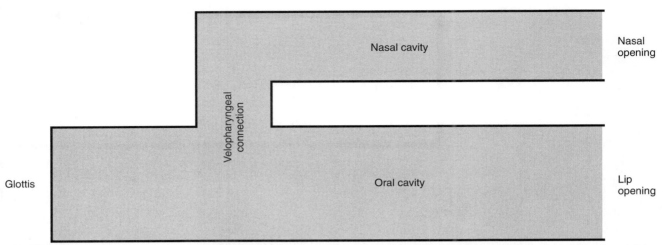

FIGURE 2-13 A schematic of the coupling of the oral and nasal cavities. (From Fucci DJ, Lass NJ: *Fundamentals of Speech Science*, 1999, Allyn & Bacon, Needham Heights, MA.)

The nasal cavity absorbs more sound energy than the oral cavity because of **antiresonances**, which suppress part of the speech spectrum. Therefore the result of nasal coupling to the oral cavity is increased damping and a reduction in amplitude of the formants.

BASIC CHARACTERISTICS OF SPEECH SOUNDS

There are four basic acoustic characteristics of speech sounds:
1. frequency
2. intensity
3. spectrum
4. duration or rate

These are the *physical* (acoustic) characteristics of speech sounds (i.e., they can be measured with appropriate instrumentation). Moreover, these physical characteristics also have perceptual correlates, which we perceive when we listen to speech sounds, but which cannot be measured. They are:
1. pitch
2. loudness
3. quality
4. perceptual judgment of duration or rate

Frequency and Pitch

The **frequency** of speech sounds is determined in the same way as the frequency of all sounds (speech and non speech): by the number of complete cycles per second of sound waves. In voice production, the fundamental frequency (f_0) is directly determined physiologically by the rate of vibration of the vocal folds and is responsible for our perception of **vocal pitch**. The faster the rate of vibra-

tion of the folds, the higher the fundamental frequency of the voice and, in turn, the higher the perceived vocal pitch. The slower the rate of vocal fold vibration, the lower the vocal fundamental frequency, and the lower the perceived vocal pitch. Thus pitch is the perceptual interpretation of frequency; in other words, we hear the pitch of a sound and not the number of cycles of vibrations (the frequency).

The frequencies important in the speech signal are within the 100 to 8000 Hz range, because this range includes the sounds with the lowest frequency (which is the average vocal fundamental frequency of the male voice of approximately 125 Hz) and those with the highest frequency (F_3 for some consonants: 8000 Hz). Thus the range of 100 to 8000 Hz includes speakers' f_0 as well as their F_1, F_2, and F_3.

Intensity and Loudness

The amount of energy in individual speech sounds is very small. However, the *range* of energy in speech sounds, from the sound with the least amount of energy to the sound with the greatest amount of energy, is very large. As a result, the intensity of sounds is expressed as a ratio rather than as an absolute magnitude. Thus acousticians have adopted the **decibel scale**, a logarithmic scale, for sound intensity. The decibel is not an absolute unit of measurement like the gram or the inch or the watt, but rather it is a ratio unit (a relative unit). It measures the intensity of sound in comparison to some other sound. In other words, it describes via logarithms (exponents) the relation (ratio) of one sound intensity to another, or to some arbitrarily chosen reference intensity. For example, when we say that the intensity of a sound is *n* dB, we mean that it is a certain number of times greater than some other intensity or some reference point. Therefore the dB refers to some intensity ratio.

Wave Complexity and Perceived Quality

It has been found that whenever complex sounds differ in perceived quality, they have different waveshapes. For example, each vowel has a different perceived quality and therefore exhibits a different waveshape from all other vowels. The differences between vowel sounds are in their quality; they are perceived as different vowels because each vowel has a characteristic waveshape which, in turn, is due to its characteristic vocal tract configuration.

Wave spectrum is the physical (acoustic) factor responsible for producing the perceptual correlate of **quality** (or in musical terms, **timbre**). **Quality** is that characteristic of complex sounds or of a voice or an instrument that distinguishes one sound from another, even if the sounds have equal pitch and loudness. For example, we can differentiate the tones of a violin versus another instrument versus human speech sounds on the basis of their characteristic qualities. Each has a different waveshape (and hence spectral) difference.

Speech sound quality (/i/ vs. /æ/ vs. /u/, etc.) is determined by the shape of the vocal tract, which in turn is determined by articulatory movements. The shape of the vocal tract affects the resonances (formants) of the vocal tract. Pure tones (partials) of the vocal fold signal that are at or near the natural or resonant (formant) frequencies of the vocal tract are resonated (amplified). It is this resonance that accounts for the quality of each speech sound.

Time, Duration, and Rate

Speech rate is commonly measured in the following units:

$$\text{Syllables per second (sps)} = \frac{\text{Number of syllables}}{\text{Total time (in sec)}}$$

$$\text{Words per second (wps)} = \frac{\text{Number of words}}{\text{Total time (in sec)}}$$

$$\text{Syllables per minute (spm)} = \frac{60 \times \text{Number of syllables}}{\text{Total time (in sec)}}$$

$$\text{Words per minute (wpm)} = \frac{60 \times \text{Number of words}}{\text{Total time (in sec)}}$$

We read aloud faster than we speak because the thinking process reduces the rate of speaking. However, in reading the same kind of thinking is not involved. Moreover, pauses are an important component of both speaking and oral reading rates. By altering pause time, we can alter overall speaking or oral reading rate as well as the perception of speech rate. There are more pauses, and pauses of longer duration, in speaking than in oral reading, which accounts for the fact that the oral reading rate is faster than the speaking rate. Moreover, this finding is also related to the thinking process involved in speaking. We use more pauses and pauses of longer duration when we think than when we are not thinking about what we will say, as is the case in oral reading.

Speaking and oral reading times are composed of two primary components: speech time and pause time.

$$\text{Total time} = \text{speech time} + \text{pause time}$$

The proportion of total time spent in pausing is called the **pause time ratio (PTR)**; it is the ratio of the time spent in pausing to the total time for the speaking or oral reading task.

$$\text{PTR} = \frac{\text{Pause time (sec)}}{\text{Total time (sec)}}$$

The proportion of total speaking or oral reading time spent in actually speaking is called the **speech time ratio (STR)**, which is the ratio of the time spent in speaking to the total time for the speaking or oral reading task.

$$\text{STR} = \frac{\text{Speech time (sec)}}{\text{Total time (sec)}}$$

also

$$\text{STR} + \text{PTR} = 1$$

and

$$1 - \text{STR} = \text{PTR}$$

and

$$1 - \text{PTR} = \text{STR}$$

Furthermore, for oral reading, pause time can be divided into intrasentence and intersentence pause times.

CONTEXTUAL EFFECTS IN SPEECH PRODUCTION

Speech is a continuously changing acoustic stream of energy produced by dynamic articulatory processes. Speech sounds are not produced in isolation but rather occur in context (conversation) and thus are influenced and altered by their neighboring sounds. Moreover, the influences that speech sounds have on neighboring sounds involve acoustic, physiologic, and perceptual aspects.

Two types of context effects (sound influence phenomena) of interest to us in speech are assimilation and coarticulation. **Assimilation** is the alteration in movement of a single articulator because of contextual effects. There are two types of assimilation: partial and complete. **Partial assimilation** involves a *phonetic* change from one allophone of a phoneme to a different allophone of the same phoneme. For example, in the production of "eat the pie," the normally linguaalveolar /t/ in *eat* is changed to a linguadental /t/. Thus the /ð/ of *the,* a linguadental fricative, has influenced the neighboring /t/ in *eat* so that the /t/ has been assimilated to the place of articulation of /ð/ (i.e., the /t/ becomes more like /ð/ in its articulation). This change is phonetic—from one allophone of /t/ (alveolar) to another allophone of /t/ (dental) of the same phoneme (i.e., no phonemic change).

Complete assimilation involves a *phonemic* change from an allophone of one phoneme to an allophone of a different phoneme. For example, in "tin cans," the lingua-alveolar /n/ in *tin* is assimilated to the place of articulation of the following linguavelar /k/ in *cans,* producing the linguavelar nasal /ŋ/.

In assimilation, the influence can be either in anticipation of the following sound (**anticipatory**, or right-to-left assimilation) or one in which an ongoing feature is continued to the next sound so that the sound is influenced by a preceding sound (**carryover**, or left-to-right assimilation). An example of **anticipatory assimilation** (when a phoneme is influenced by a following phoneme) occurs in the word *blank* [blæŋk] because the [n] is changed to [ŋ] in anticipation of the following [k]. Thus velar-palatal placement is extended to the normally alveolar /n/ in *blank,* producing [blæŋk] (which assimilates the nasal to the more posterior /k/ place of articulation).

An example of **carryover assimilation** occurs in plural endings after voiced consonants. The /s/ in *caps* remains an [s], but the /s/ in *cabs* changes to [z] because the voicing in /b/ is carried over to the /s/ and thereby converts it to [z]. The changes associated with the contextual effects of assimilation include acoustic (spectrographic), physiologic (muscle activity), and perceptual features.

Coarticulation, a term coined by Sven Öhman of Sweden, is the phenomenon of two articulators moving at the same time for the production of different phonemes. An example of coarticulation occurs in the production of the word *two,* in which the speaker rounds the lips for [u] while the tongue is active for the production of [t]. Therefore the lips and tongue are moving simultaneously for different phonemes. Coarticulation has been reported in acoustical (spectrographic), movement (x-ray), and muscle action (electromyographic) studies. For example, it has been discovered that liprounding for [u] can start at the beginning of a consonant-consonant-vowel (CCV)

syllable if there is no articulatory movement competitive to it (i.e., if none of the intervening sounds require a movement antagonistic to [u]). For example, when the initial sound in a word is a nasal that involves tongue movement (as the /n/ in the word *not*), then the mandible is free to lower and produce the [a] at the same time as the tongue movement. But if the initial sound is a plosive (e.g., the plosive /t/ in *top* or *tap*), then the mandible has to wait until the alveolar closure for [t] before it can start moving toward the vowel. Because plosives require high intraoral breath pressure behind the point of closure and nasals do not, premature jaw lowering after a plosive threatens the needed pressure for the plosive, and therefore coarticulation in this case does not occur.

In conversational speech, coarticulation and assimilation of one articulatory movement to another (called **parallel processing**) is very common and it is this combination that makes speech transmission both rapid and efficient. All sound influences show that speech is not produced as a series of isolated, independent sounds, like beads of isolated phones put together on a string, one phone after another. For example, the production of the word *pie* is never accomplished by saying [p] and then quickly producing [aI]. If the phonemes are produced independently of each other, no matter how rapidly the [aI] follows the [p], the utterance will not be heard as *pie*. Why? Because speakers coarticulate; in other words, they produce more than one phoneme at the same time. While the lips are closed for the bilabial [p] in *pie,* the tongue is lowering for the beginning of the diphthong [aI], and while the lips are opening to release the burst in [p], the tongue is moving forward (fronting) and elevating for the production of the off-glide of the diphthong [aI]. Thus phonemes do not exist as independent units, but rather overlap and merge into one continuously changing stream of sound.

REVIEW EXERCISES

TRUE-FALSE

1. The vocal fundamental frequency is the pure tone with the lowest amplitude in the signal produced by the vocal folds.

2. The vocal tract is an air-filled tube and therefore can act as a resonator.

3. When the sound wave produced by the vocal folds is transmitted through the vocal tract, the tract will respond better to those components of the vocal fold signal that are at, or near, its natural (resonant) frequencies.

4. The human vocal tract is a multiply resonant tube.

5. Each vowel sound has its own unique set of formant frequencies.

6. For front vowels, as the cross-sectional area (radius, size) of the maximum constriction of the vocal tract increases, F_1 decreases.

7. In the speech production process, the generator system is responsible for producing the fundamental frequency and harmonics of the voice.

8. It is possible to alter vocal fundamental frequency without altering the characteristic quality of a vowel sound.

9. The human vocal tract is considered to be analogous to a tube open at both ends.

10. Usually females have higher formant frequencies than males because they usually have shorter vocal tracts.

11. The acoustic energy in an individual speech sound is very small.

12. Speech sound quality (/i/ vs. /æ/ vs. /u/, etc.) is determined by the shape of the vocal tract, which in turn is determined by movements of the articulators.

13. Complex sounds with different waveshapes have different perceived quality.

14. Speech sounds are not produced in isolation but rather occur in context (conversation) and thus are influenced by their neighboring sounds.

15. Partial assimilation involves a phonemic change from an allophone of one phoneme to an allophone of a different phoneme.

16. Anticipatory assimilation is one in which an ongoing feature is continued to the next sound so that the sound is influenced by a preceding sound.

17. Coarticulation is the phenomenon of two articulators moving, one after the other in time, for different phonemes.

18. Speech is produced as a series of isolated, independent sounds, like beads of isolated phones put together on a string, one phone after another.

19. In conversational speech phonemes do not exist as independent units, but rather overlap and merge into one continuously changing stream of sound.

20. Coarticulation occurs in the production of the word *top*, with the mandible moving for the vowel at the same time as the tongue is moving for the production of the linguaalveolar /t/.

FILL IN THE BLANK

1. The parts of the body involved in speech production include the _____, _____, _____, _____, _____, and _____.

2. The theory proposed by Dr. Gunnar Fant to explain how sound produced by the vocal folds is modified by the acoustic properties of the vocal tract is called the _____ theory.

3. The _____ is the portion of the speech production mechanism that extends from the glottis to the lips and includes the larynx, pharynx, oral cavity, and nasal cavity.

4. Stopping the flow of air completely, but only momentarily, via the blocking of the vocal tract with the tongue or lips and then suddenly releasing the air pressure built up behind this air blockage produces speech sounds classified as _____.

5. The natural (resonant) frequencies of the human vocal tract are called _____.

6. The peaks in the spectra of vowels, which are the regions in which the frequency components are relatively high in amplitude, correspond to the _____ of the vocal tract.

7. The quantitative values of the formant frequencies of vowels depend on three physiologic factors:
   a. _____
   b. _____
   c. _____

8. In the speech production process, the resonator system is responsible for determining the _____ of the vocal tract.

9. The perceptual correlate of vocal fundamental frequency is vocal _____.

10. The intensity of speech sounds is frequently expressed as a ratio rather than an absolute magnitude by using the _____ scale.

11. _____ is that characteristic of complex sounds (like those produced by the voice or musical instruments) that distinguishes one sound from another, even if the sounds have equal pitch and loudness.

12. In "eat the vegetables," the normally linguaalveolar /t/ in *eat* is changed to a _____ /t/ so that the /t/ is assimilated to the place of articulation of /ð/ in *the* (i.e., the /t/ becomes more like /ð/ in its articulation).

13. In the word *blank* the [n] is changed to /ŋ/ in anticipation of the following [k]. This is an example of _____ assimilation.

14. The /s/ in *taps* remains an [s], but the /s/ in *tabs* changes to [z]. This is an example of _____ assimilation.

15. In the production of the word *two*, the speaker rounds the lips for [u] while the tongue is active for the production of [t]. This phenomenon is called _____.

MULTIPLE CHOICE

1. The signal produced by the vocal folds can be characterized acoustically as a _____ signal.
   a. simple periodic
   b. complex aperiodic
   c. simple aperiodic
   d. complex quasiperiodic
   e. none of the above

2. A method for making the airstream from the lungs audible involves constricting the vocal tract at some point along its length, with the airstream passing through the constriction becoming turbulent. This method is responsible for producing speech sounds classified as:
   a. plosives
   b. diphthongs
   c. vowels
   d. fricatives
   e. none of the above

3. For front vowels, the chief cause of variation in F_1 is:
   a. size (radius, cross-sectional area) of maximum constriction in oral cavity
   b. position of maximum constriction relative to its distance from the glottis
   c. liprounding
   d. all of the above
   e. none of the above

4. For back vowels, the chief cause of variation in F_1 is:
   a. size (radius, cross-sectional area) of maximum constriction in oral cavity
   b. position of point of maximum constriction relative to its distance from the glottis
   c. liprounding
   d. all of the above
   e. none of the above

5. For a tube open at one end and closed at the other end, and of uniform cross-sectional dimensions throughout its length, the lowest resonant frequency is equal to the frequency of a sound wave whose wavelength (λ) is _____ times the length of the tube.
   a. 10
   b. 2
   c. 5
   d. 20
   e. none of the above

6. Coupling the oral cavity to the nasal cavity results in:
   a. increased vocal fundamental frequency
   b. increased vocal amplitude
   c. increased vocal duration
   d. all of the above
   e. none of the above

7. The perceptual correlate of the spectrum of the voice is vocal:
   a. pitch
   b. loudness
   c. rate
   d. quality
   e. none of the above

8. For speech comprehension purposes, the most important range of frequencies in the speech signal is _____ Hz.
   a. 20-20,000
   b. 250-8000
   c. 500-2000
   d. 100-8000
   e. 10-20,000

COMPUTATIONAL PROBLEMS

1. For a tube open at one end and closed at the other end, of uniform cross-sectional dimensions throughout its length, the *nth* resonant frequency is equal to the frequency of a sound wave whose wavelength (λ) is _____ times the length of the tube.
   a. 4/n-1
   b. 2/4n-1
   c. n/4-1
   d. 4/2n-1
   e. none of the above

2. The third formant frequency of the average adult female vocal tract is _____ Hz.
   a. 12
   b. 2500
   c. 2833
   d. 567
   e. 94

3. The tenth formant frequency of the average adult male vocal tract is _____ Hz.
   a. 9497
   b. 500
   c. 10,767
   d. 95
   e. 567

4. If a speaker reads aloud a 300-word, 750-syllable reading passage in 2 minutes, her/his reading rate is _____ wps.
   a. 150
   b. 2.5
   c. 0.4
   d. 6.25
   e. none of the above

5. If a speaker reads aloud a 500-word, 1000-syllable reading passage in 150 seconds, his/her reading rate is _____ wpm.
   a. 200
   b. 3.3
   c. 6.7
   d. 150
   e. 400

6. If a speaker reads aloud a 520-word, 1000-syllable passage in 660 seconds, her/his reading rate is _____ spm.
   a. 91
   b. 5454
   c. 2836
   d. 47
   e. none of the above

7. Given the following information about a speaker's reading of a prose passage:

1000 words

1300 syllables

speech time = 200 seconds

intrasentence pause time = 70 seconds

intersentence pause time = 30 seconds

This speaker's syllables per second rate is _____ sps.

This speaker's words per second rate is _____ wps.

This speaker's speech-time ratio is _____.

This speaker's pause-time ratio is _____.

APPLICATION EXERCISES

1. Describe the acoustic theory (source-filter theory) and discuss its importance in understanding the acoustics of speech production.

2. What are the clinical implications and applications associated with the fact that each different configuration of the vocal tract has its own unique set of formant frequencies?

3. Discuss the clinical implications and applications of the fact that the generator and resonator systems involved in speech production operate independently of each other.

4. Discuss the clinical applications and implications of the physiological and acoustic differences between the fundamental and formant frequencies of: (a) female vs. male speakers and (b) children vs. adult speakers.

5. Discuss the clinical applications and implications of the presence of antiresonances when there is a coupling of the oral and nasal cavities.

6. Discuss the difference between *voice quality* and *vowel quality* and the clinical relevance of this difference.

7. Discuss the clinical implications and applications of the fact that in speech production and speech perception, pause time is an important component in overall speaking time.

8. Discuss the clinical importance of the contextual effects (sound influence phenomena) of assimilation and coarticulation in the diagnosis and treatment of articulation disorders.

Anatomy and Physiology

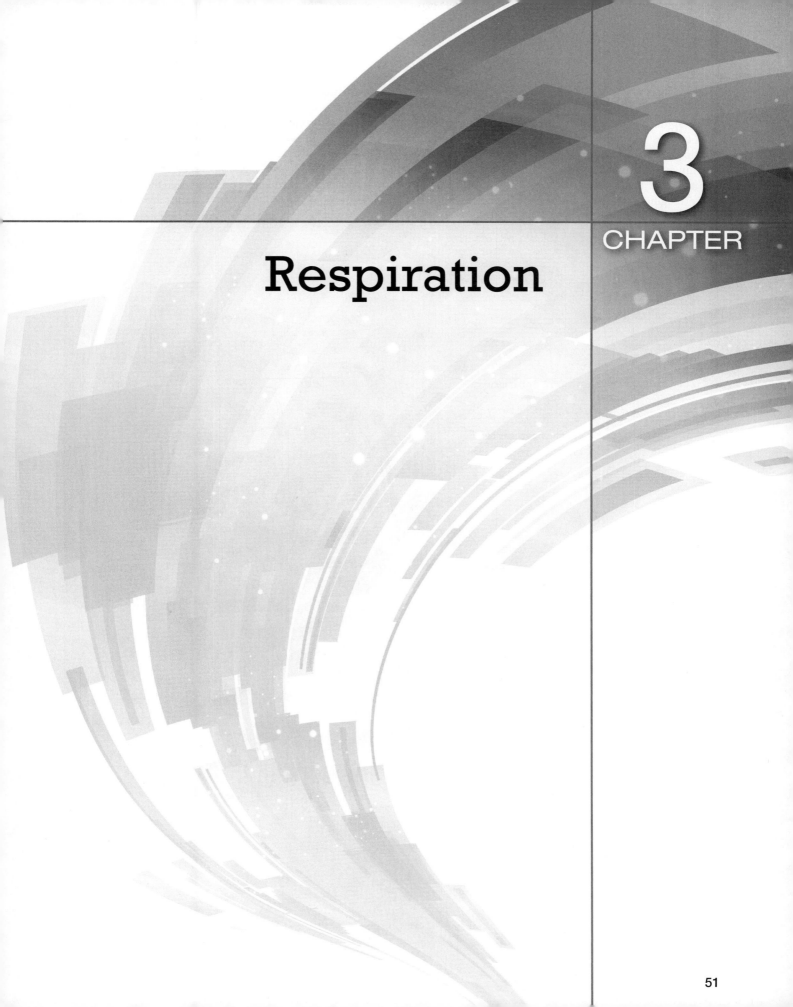

Respiration

RESPIRATORY TRACT

The respiratory tract includes the nasal, oral, and pharyngeal cavities, larynx, trachea, and lungs, thus forming a continuous open passageway from the atmospheric air to the lungs (Figure 3-1). Air passes to and from the lungs through the **trachea**, an unpaired structure composed of cartilaginous rings connected by membranes. At its lower end it bifurcates to yield a right and left **mainstem**

bronchus, with each mainstem bronchus entering the respective lung (Figures 3-1 and 3-2). Once they enter the lung, the bronchi experience more than 20 divisions that end in an air sac containing **pulmonary alveoli**, small pits lying very near blood vessels. Each alveolus shares a wall with the blood vessels; gases (oxygen and carbon dioxide) are exchanged through this wall between the lung spaces and the transporting blood. The two **lungs** are air-filled structures divided into **lobes**, with three lobes in the right lung

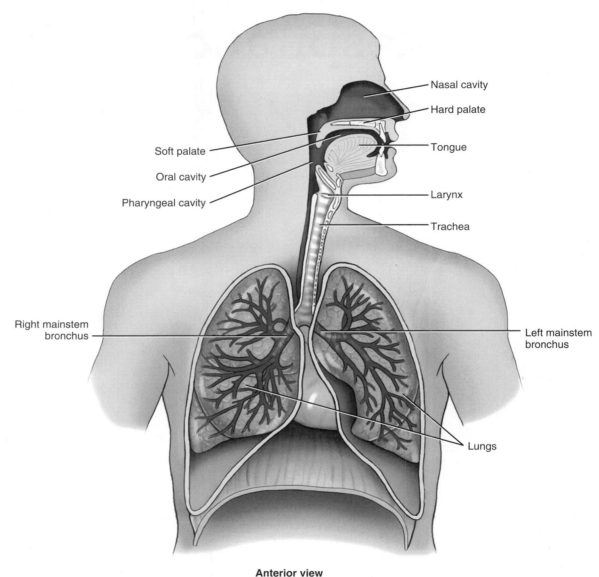

Anterior view

FIGURE 3-1 Respiratory tract.

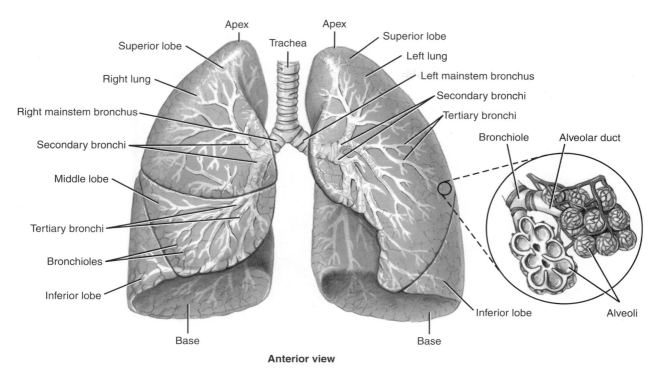

FIGURE 3-2 Trachea, bronchi, and lungs.

but only two in the left lung because of the presence of the heart and other mediastinal contents.

Respiration involves the inhalation of air to provide oxygen to the body's tissues and the exhalation of air for the removal of carbon dioxide. For speech purposes, respiration is a physical process that involves pumping air into the lungs and exhaling air to speak; the movement of air out of the lungs is transformed into acoustical energy. Exhalation of air for speech purposes is thought to be an overlaid function whereby humans have learned to adapt a system, which is biologically intended to preserve the body's tissues, for speech production purposes. Respiration provides the energy source needed to produce speech sounds.

BONY SKELETAL FRAMEWORK

The bony skeletal framework for respiration consists of the **vertebral column**, **rib cage**, **pectoral girdle**, and **pelvic girdle**. The vertebral column (Figures 3-3 and 3-4) consists of 32 or 33 individual vertebrae that are joined together by intervertebral cartilaginous discs, including seven **cervical vertebrae** in the neck region, twelve **thoracic vertebrae** in the chest region, five **lumbar vertebrae** in the back region, five **sacral vertebrae** (fused together into one bone, the **sacrum**) in the portion of the pelvic (hip) region, and three or four **coccygeal vertebrae** (fused into one **coccyx**) at the lower end of the vertebral column. The 12 thoracic vertebrae serve as the posterior attachments for the 12

Text cont'd on p. 56

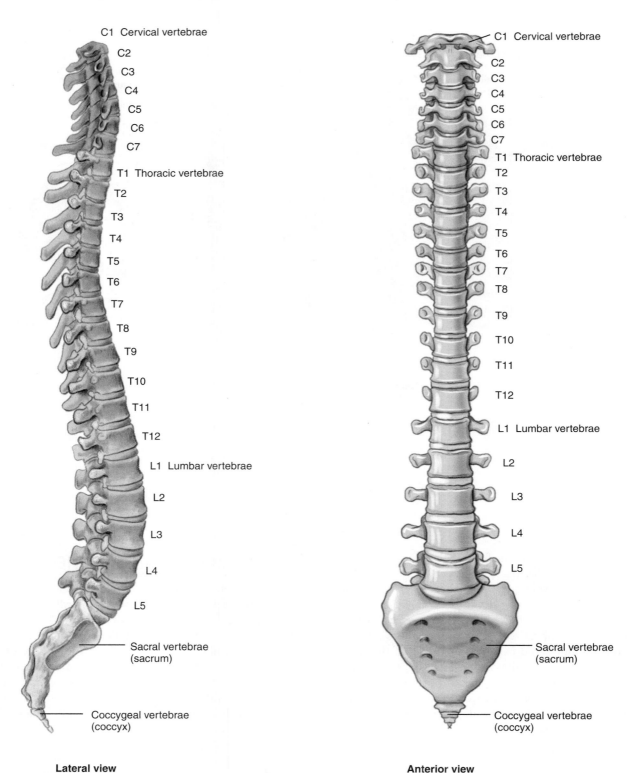

Lateral view

Anterior view

FIGURE 3-3 Vertebral column.

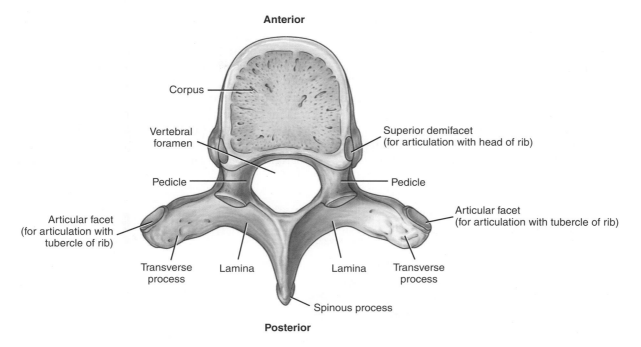

Anterior

Corpus

Vertebral foramen

Superior demifacet
(for articulation with head of rib)

Pedicle

Pedicle

Articular facet
(for articulation with
tubercle of rib)

Articular facet
(for articulation with tubercle of rib)

Transverse
process

Lamina

Lamina

Transverse
process

Spinous process

Posterior

Superior view

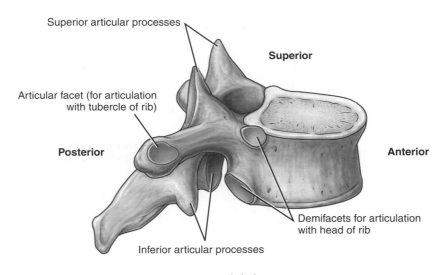

Superior articular processes

Superior

Articular facet (for articulation
with tubercle of rib)

Posterior

Anterior

Demifacets for articulation
with head of rib

Inferior articular processes

Inferior

Lateral view

FIGURE 3-4 Thoracic vertebra.

pairs of ribs. The **rib cage** includes 12 pairs of ribs attached posteriorly to the 12 thoracic vertebrae and anteriorly to the **sternum** (breastbone) (Figures 3-5, 3-6, and 3-7), an unpaired segmented bone in the midline on the superior-anterior thoracic wall that protects the contents of the thorax. The sternum consists of the **manubrium**, the most superior portion; the **corpus**, the bulk of the sternum; and the **ensiform** (or **xiphoid**) **process**, the most inferior portion. The first seven ribs are attached directly to the sternum; hence they are called **vertebrosternal** (or **true**) **ribs**. Ribs 8,

9, and 10 are attached to the sternum indirectly through a common costal cartilage; they are called **vertebrochondral** (or **false**) **ribs**. The remaining two ribs, ribs 11 and 12, are not connected to the sternum and their ventral ends are imbedded in the abdominal musculature; they are referred to as **floating ribs**.

The ribs vary in size, getting progressively larger from ribs 1 through 7 and then progressively smaller from ribs 8 through 12, which gives the thoracic framework a barrel-like shape. The typical rib consists of the **head** (the

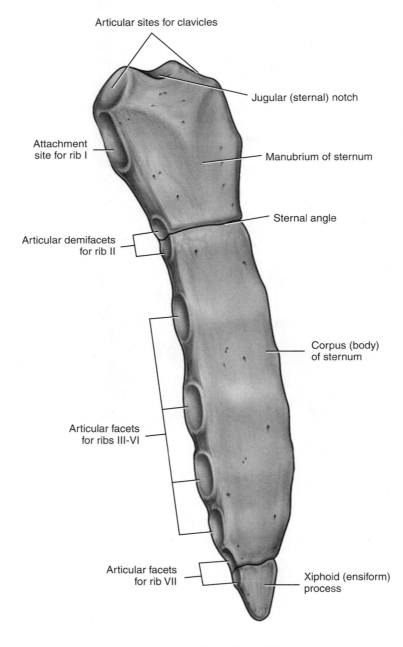

Anterolateral view

FIGURE 3-5 Sternum.

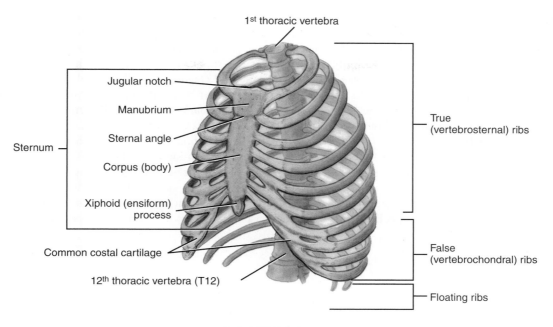

1st thoracic vertebra

Jugular notch

Manubrium

Sternal angle

Sternum

Corpus (body)

Xiphoid (ensiform) process

True (vertebrosternal) ribs

Common costal cartilage

False (vertebrochondral) ribs

12th thoracic vertebra (T12)

Floating ribs

Anterolateral view

FIGURE 3-6 Rib cage.

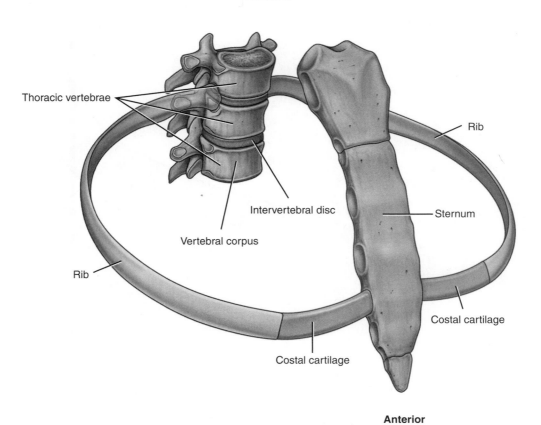

Posterior

Thoracic vertebrae

Rib

Intervertebral disc

Sternum

Vertebral corpus

Rib

Costal cartilage

Costal cartilage

Anterior

Anterolateral view

FIGURE 3-7 Anterior and posterior attachments of a rib.

most posterior portion of the rib that attaches to the corpus of each thoracic vertebra); the **shaft** (or **body**), which composes the bulk of the rib; the **neck** (the constricted portion that separates the head from the shaft of the rib); the **tubercle** (a small rounded projection at the juncture of the neck and shaft that articulates with the transverse process of each thoracic vertebra); and the **angle** of the rib, the point where the rib changes direction to curve anteriorly and then medially toward the anterior midline of the thorax. The twist of the ribs, which permits them to move outward when elevated, occurs at their angle (Figure 3-8).

The **pectoral** (shoulder) **girdle** is a supportive structure that provides the attachment of the upper limbs to the torso (trunk) of the body. It includes two structures: the **clavicle** (collarbone) and **scapula** (shoulder blade) (Figure 3-9).

The **pelvic girdle** consists of paired **coxal** (hip) **bones**; it is a supportive structure to which the lower limbs are attached (Figure 3-10). The coxal bones are composed of three lesser bones: the **ilium**, **ischium**, and **pubis**. Important landmarks include the **iliac crest**, **acetabulum** (serves as a joint socket for the reception of the head of the **femur** [upper leg bone]), **ischial tuberosity** (a rounded projection representing the end of the ischium), **pubic symphysis** (a line representing the meeting of the two pubic bones, one from one side of the body with the other from the other side of the body), and **inguinal ligament** (a ligament extending from the pubic symphysis to the iliac crest).

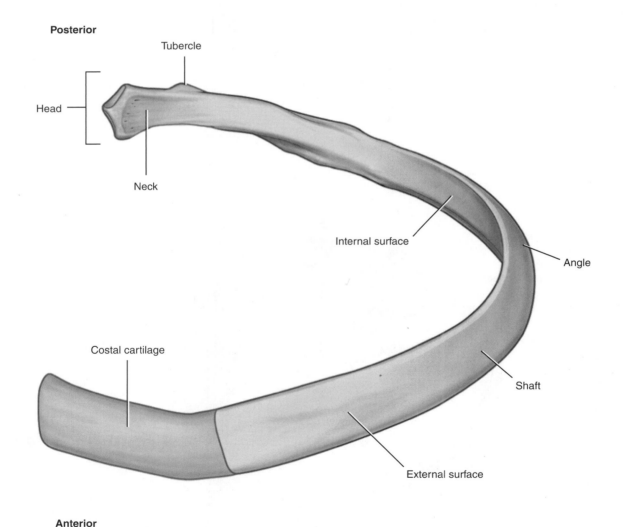

FIGURE 3-8 Rib.

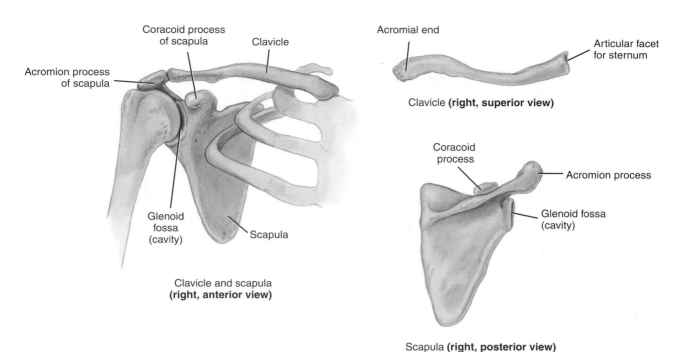

FIGURE 3-9 Pectoral girdle: clavicle and scapula.

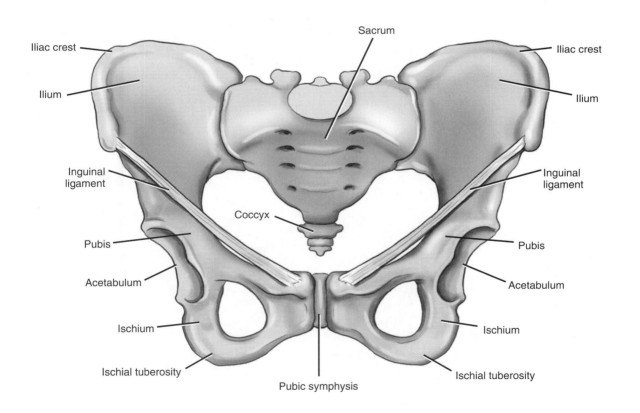

Anterior view

FIGURE 3-10 Pelvic girdle: ilium, ischium, and pubis bones.

MUSCLES

Muscles play a major role in the respiratory process. The specific number of muscles involved depends on the demand that the body places on the pumping action involved in respiration. During the inhalation phase of respiration, muscles move the ribs and sternum (to which the ribs are attached) upward and outward, which expands the volume of the thoracic cavity, creating a negative pressure relative to atmospheric pressure. Therefore air rushes into the lungs to equalize atmospheric pressure and thoracic cavity pressure.

The inhalation phase is followed by the exhalation phase. Although no muscle contraction is involved in passive exhalation, there are nonmuscular forces at work:

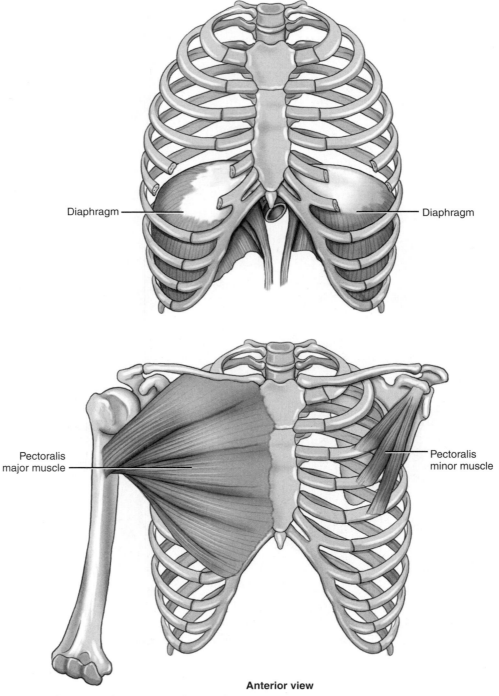

Anterior view

FIGURE 3-11 Thoracic muscles: diaphragm, pectoralis major, pectoral minor.

elasticity (of muscles, lung tissue, ribs, costal cartilages, and viscera underlying the diaphragm), and **gravitational forces** (the effects of gravity on the body's skeleton). During forced exhalation, the ribs and sternum are lowered and pulled inward, creating decreased volume and therefore increased pressure in the thoracic cavity relative to the outside atmosphere, which forces air out of the lungs and into the atmosphere.

Although there is some disagreement as to the importance and function of specific muscles in the respiratory process, those that appear to be of importance in elevating the ribs and allowing air to rush into the lungs during inhalation are the thoracic muscles (Figures 3-11 and 3-12), neck muscles (Figures 3-13 and 3-14), and some back muscles (Figures 3-15 and 3-16). The primary muscles involved in lowering the ribs and allowing air to rush out of the lungs during exhalation are abdominal muscles (Figure 3-17) with assistance from some back and thoracic muscles.

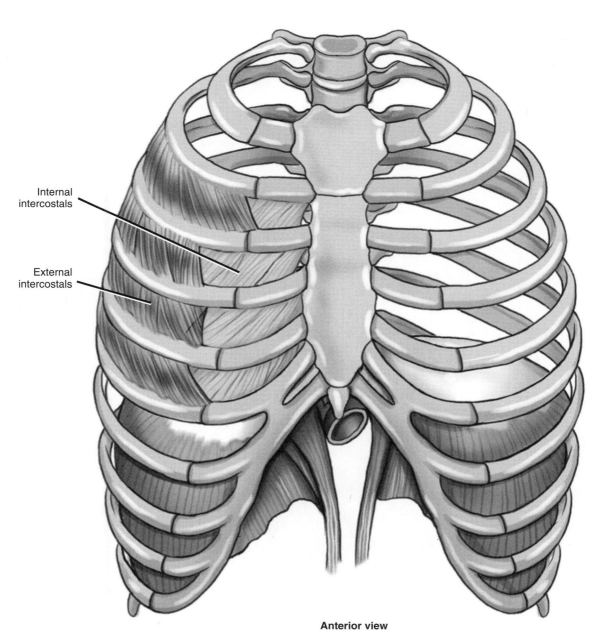

Internal
intercostals

External
intercostals

Anterior view

FIGURE 3-12 Thoracic muscles: internal and external intercostals.

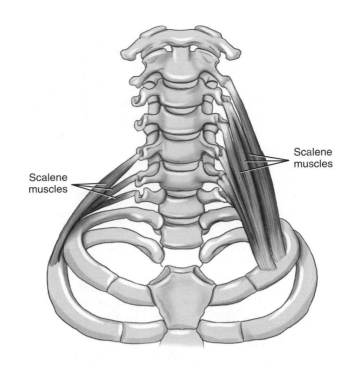

Anterior view

FIGURE 3-13 Neck muscles: scalene.

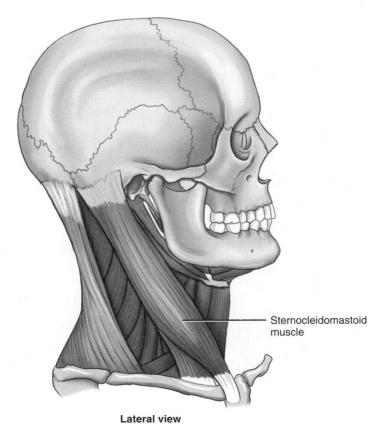

Lateral view

FIGURE 3-14 Neck muscle: sternocleidomastoid.

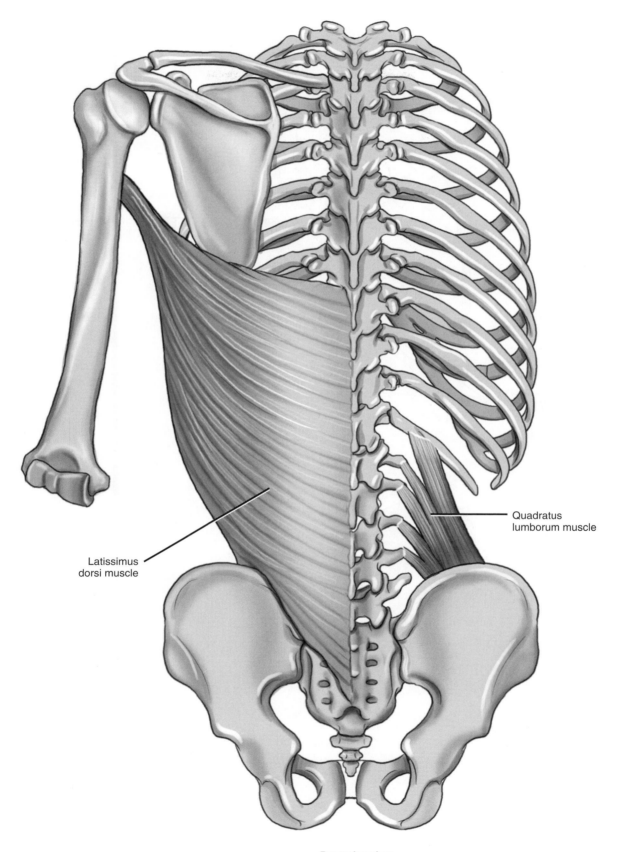

Quadratus
lumborum muscle

Latissimus
dorsi muscle

Posterior view

FIGURE 3-15 Back muscles: latissimus dorsi and quadratus lumborum.

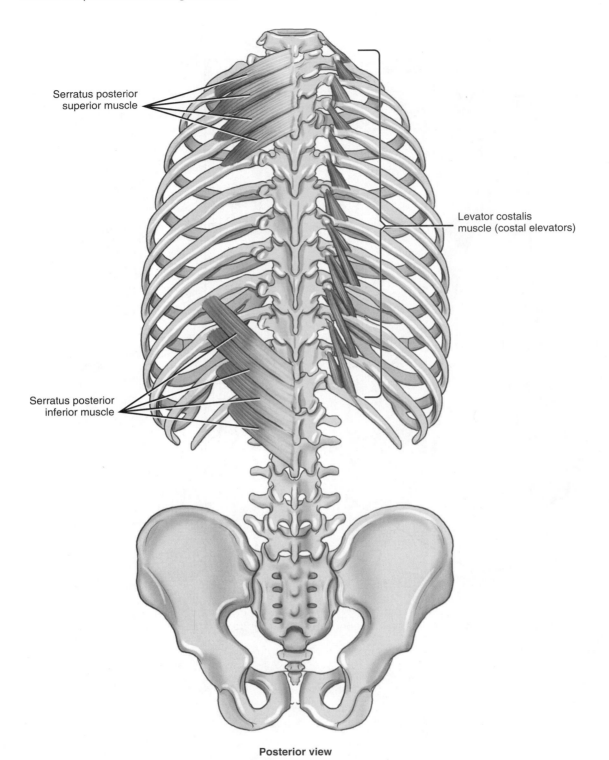

Serratus posterior
superior muscle

Levator costalis
muscle (costal elevators)

Serratus posterior
inferior muscle

Posterior view

FIGURE 3-16 Back muscles: serratus posterior superior, serratus poster inferior, and levator costalis.

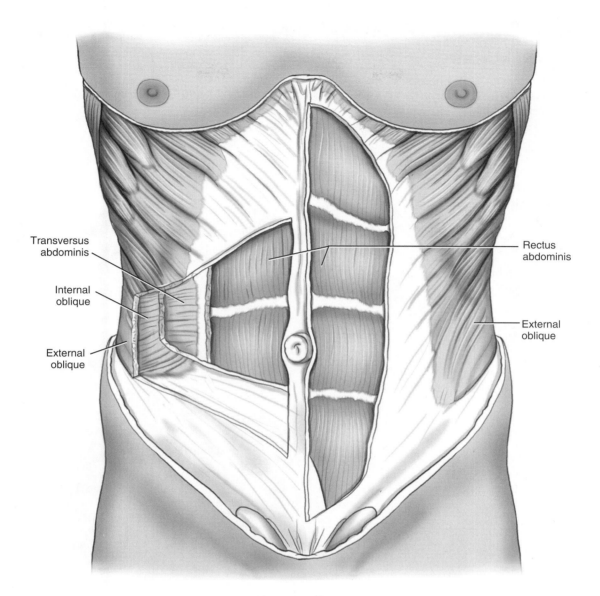

Transversus abdominis

Internal oblique

External oblique

Rectus abdominis

External oblique

Anterior view

FIGURE 3-17 Abdominal muscles: transversus abdominis, rectus abdominis, internal oblique, and external oblique.

REVIEW EXERCISES

ANATOMY EXERCISES

LEVEL 1

In the illustrations in Level 1, (a) identify each anatomical structure, and (b) identify each listed part by drawing a line to each part and labeling it.

1. _____

    nasal cavity

    oral cavity

    pharyngeal cavity

    larynx

    trachea

    right mainstream bronchus

    left mainstream bronchus

    lungs

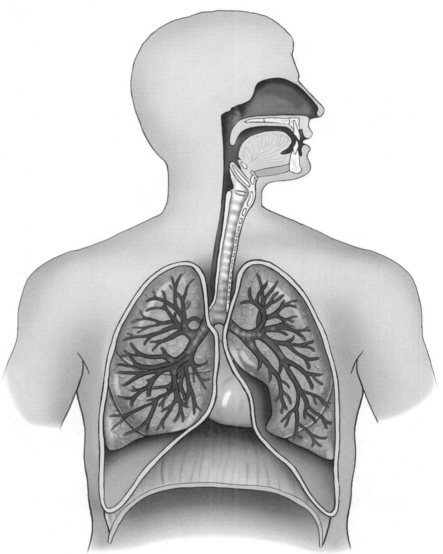

2. _____

superior lobe

middle lobe

inferior lobe

apex

base

right mainstem bronchus

left mainstem bronchus

secondary bronchi

tertiary bronchi

bronchioles

alveoli

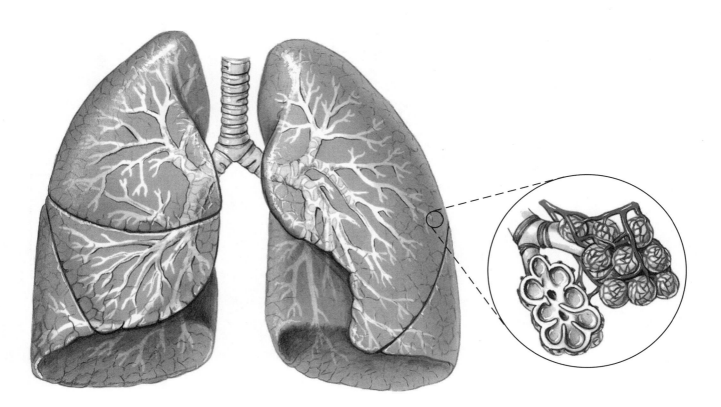

3. _____

cervical vertebrae

thoracic vertebrae

lumbar vertebrae

sacral vertebrae (sacrum)

coccygeal vertebrae (coccyx)

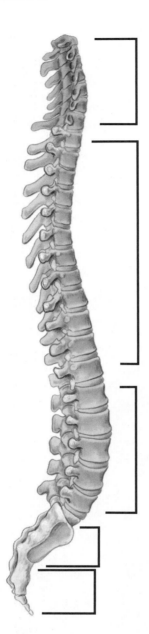

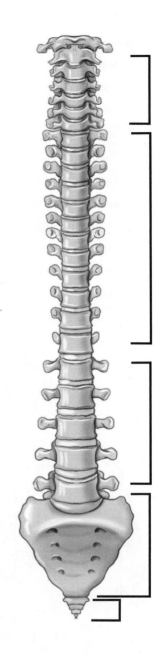

4. _____

corpus (body)

foramen

pedicle

lamina

transverse processes

spinous process

superior articular processes

articular facets

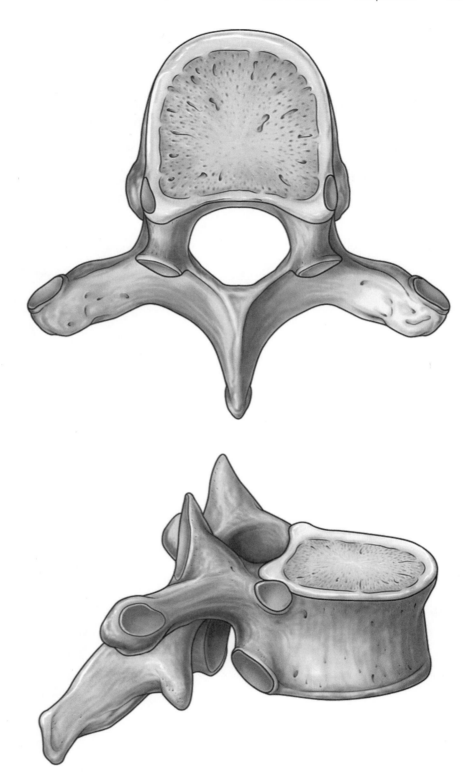

5. _____

   manubrium

   corpus (body)

   xiphoid (ensiform) process

   angle

   jugular notch

   articular facets

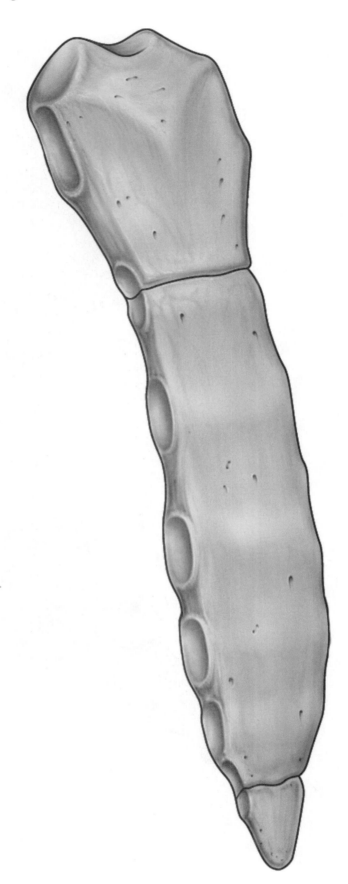

6. _____

  ribs

  sternum

  common costal cartilage

  thoracic vertebrae

  vertebrosternal (true) ribs

  vertebrochondral (false) ribs

  floating ribs

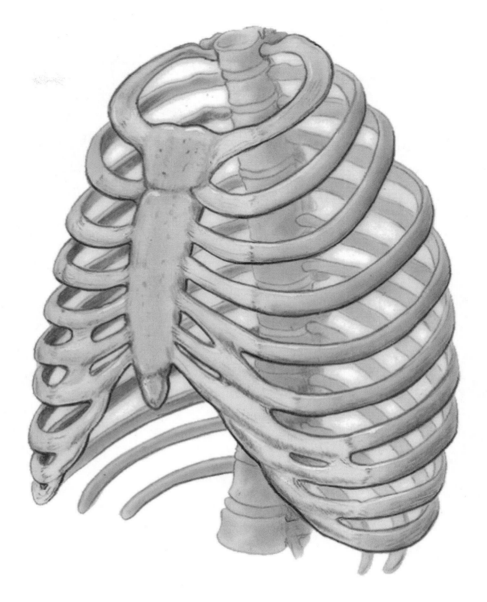

7. _____

    rib

    thoracic vertabrae

    sternum

    coastal cartilage

    intervertebral disc

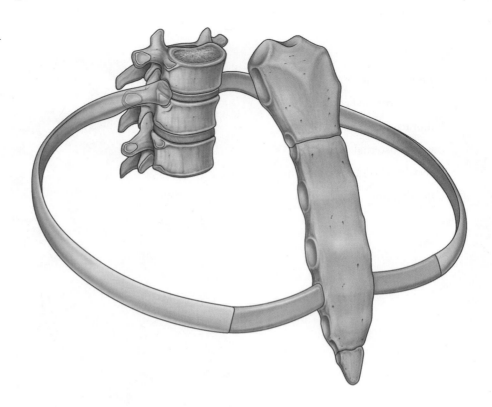

8. _____

head

shaft (body)

neck

tubercle

angle

costal cartilage

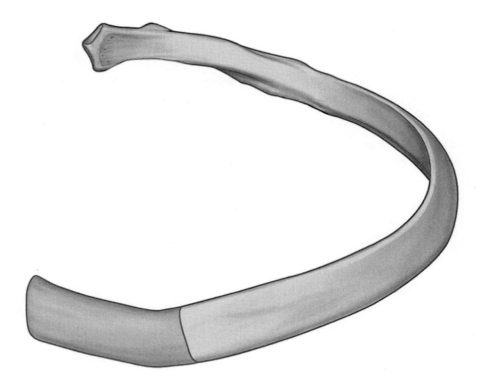

9. _____

clavicle

scapula

acromion process

coracoid process

glenoid fossa

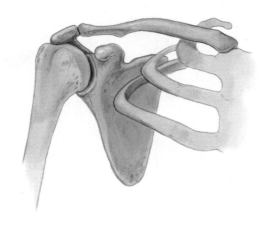
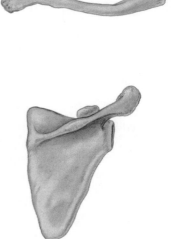

10. _____

ilium

ischium

pubis

iliac crest

acetabulum

ischial tuberosity

pubic symphysis

inguinal ligament

sacrum

coccyx

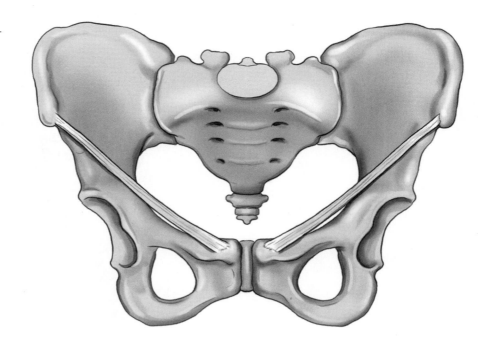

11. _____

diaphragm

pectoralis major

pectoralis minor

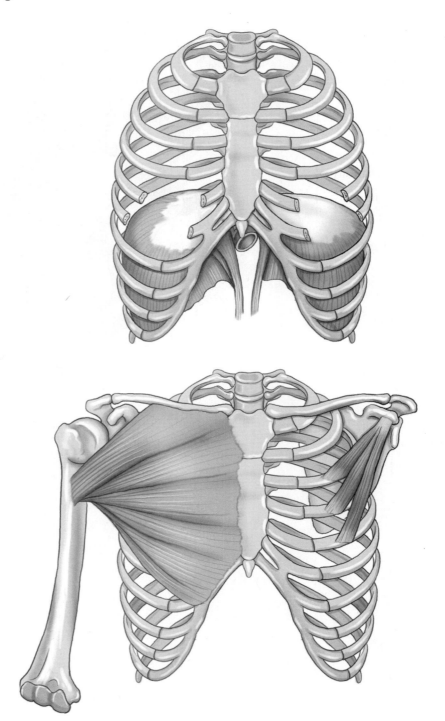

12. _____

internal intercostals

external intercostals

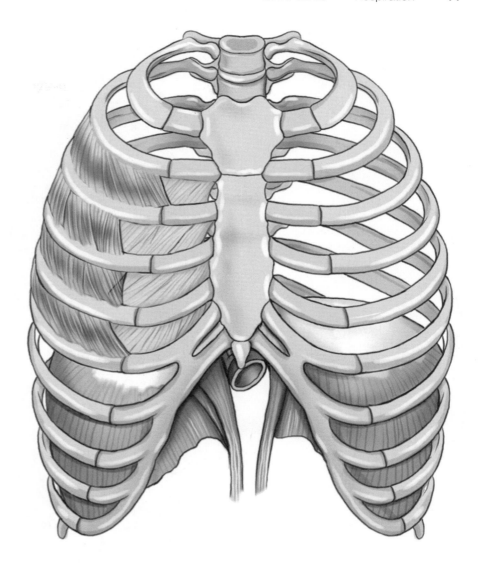

13. _____

scaleni

sternocleidomastoid

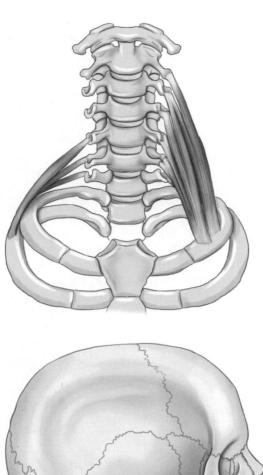

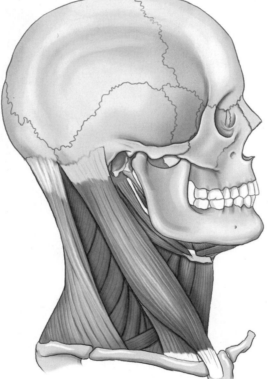

14. _____

latissimus dorsi

quadratus lumborum

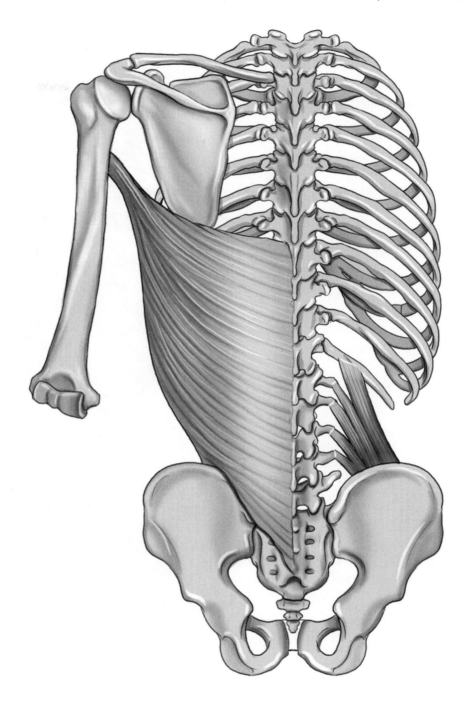

15. _____

serratus posterior superior

serratus posterior inferior

levator costalis

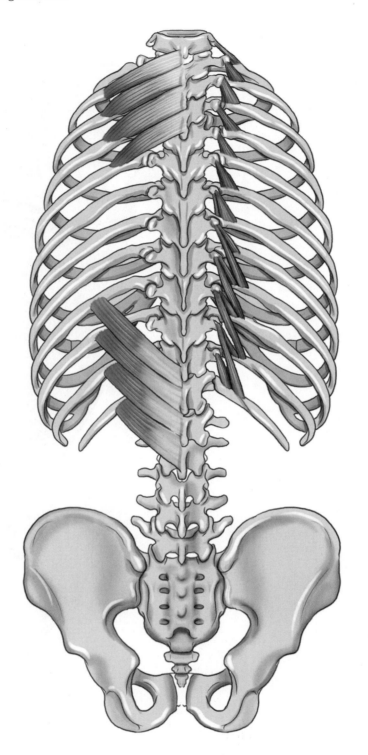

16. _____

internal oblique

external oblique

rectus abdominis

transversus abdominis

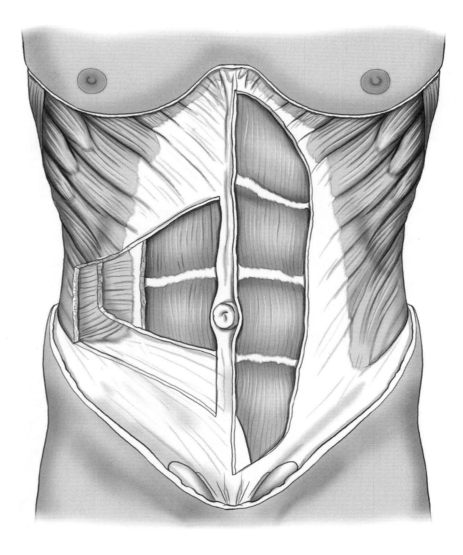

LEVEL 2

In Level 2, identify each anatomical part indicated by lines in the illustrations below.

1.

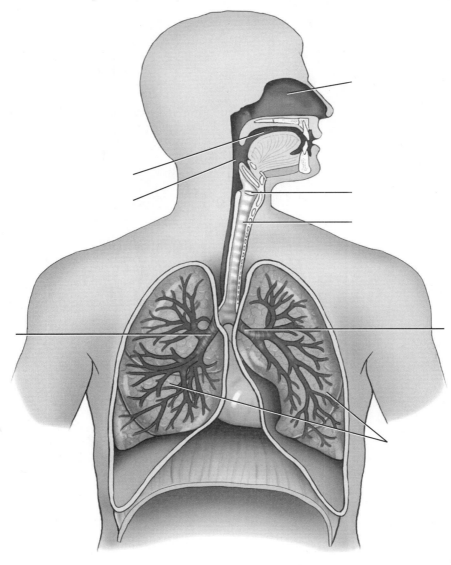

2.

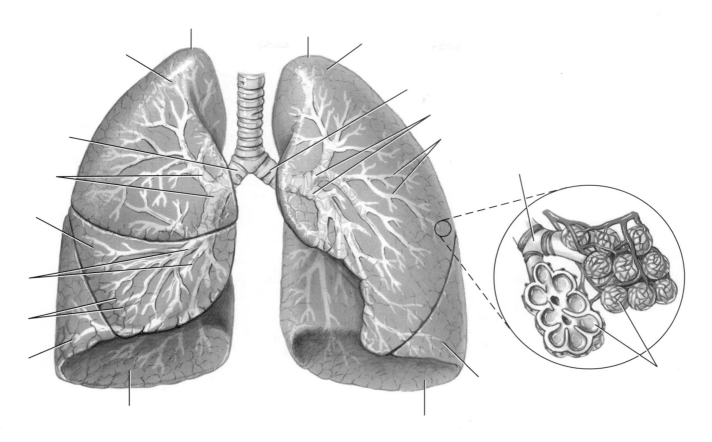

3.

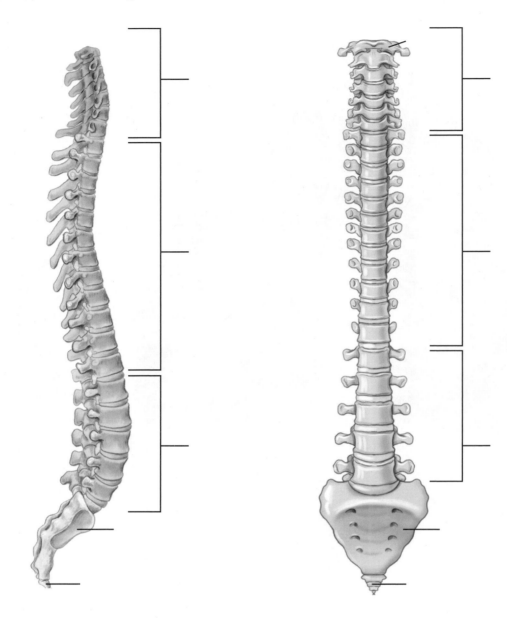

4.

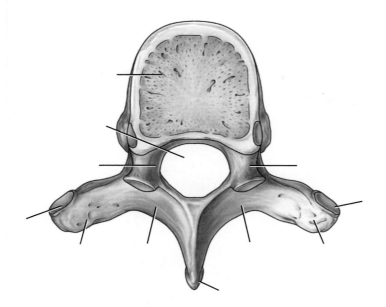

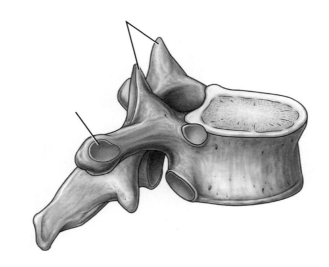

5.

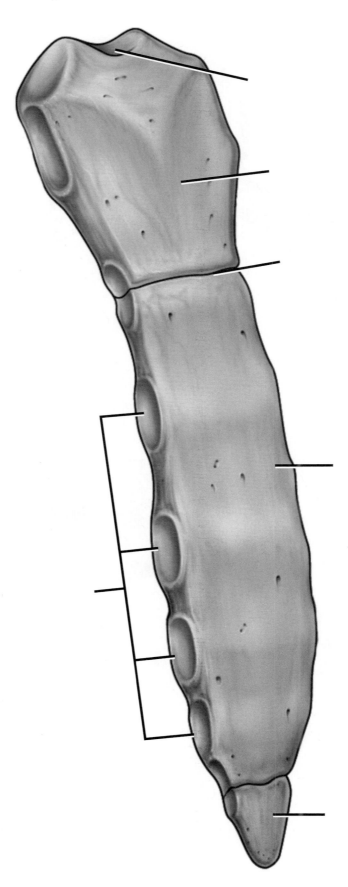

6.

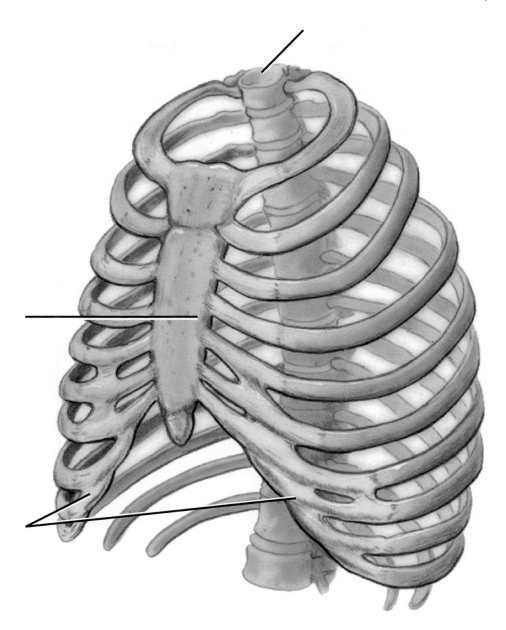

7.

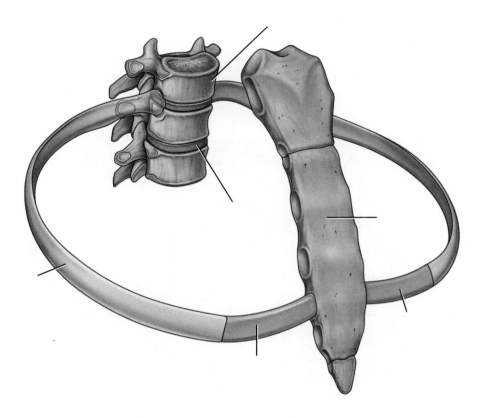

8.

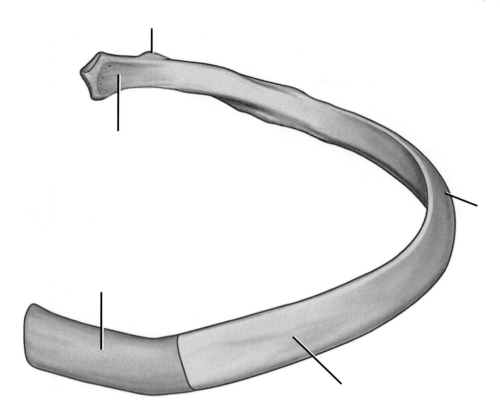

9.

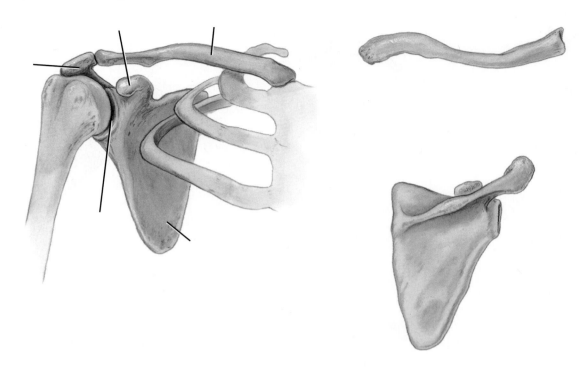

10.

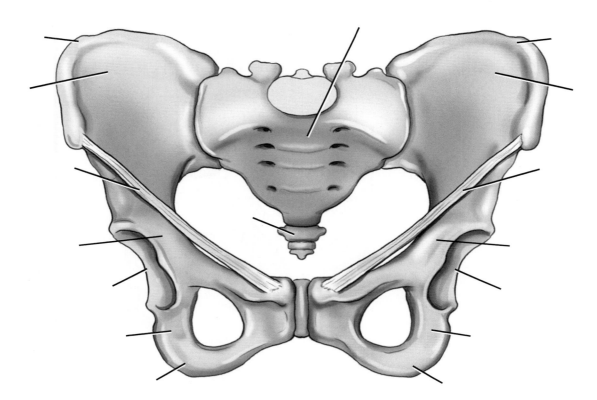

11.

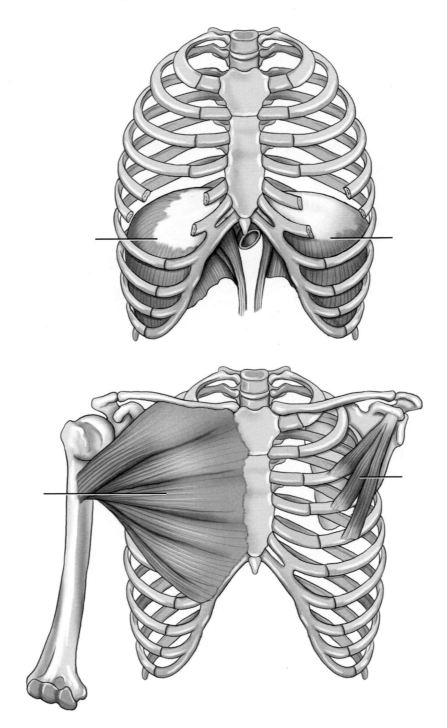

12.

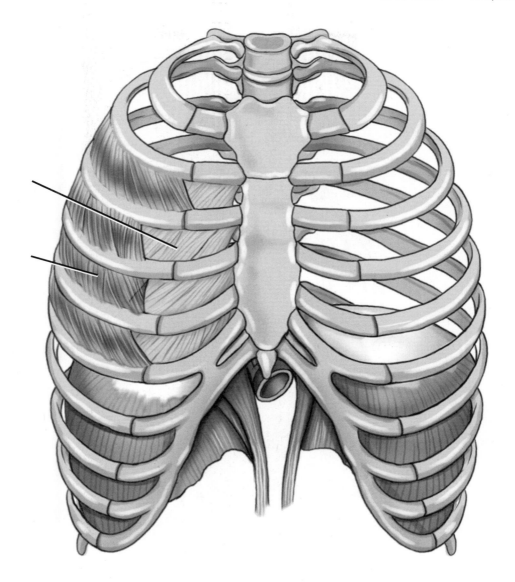

13.

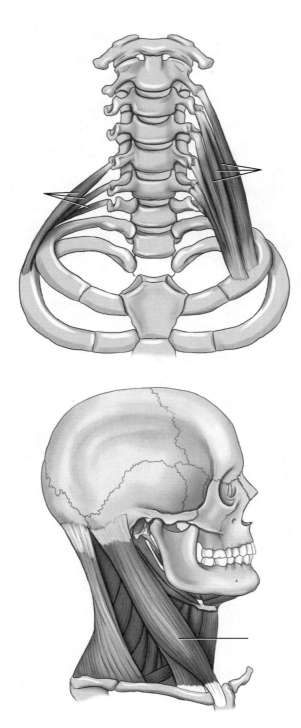

14.

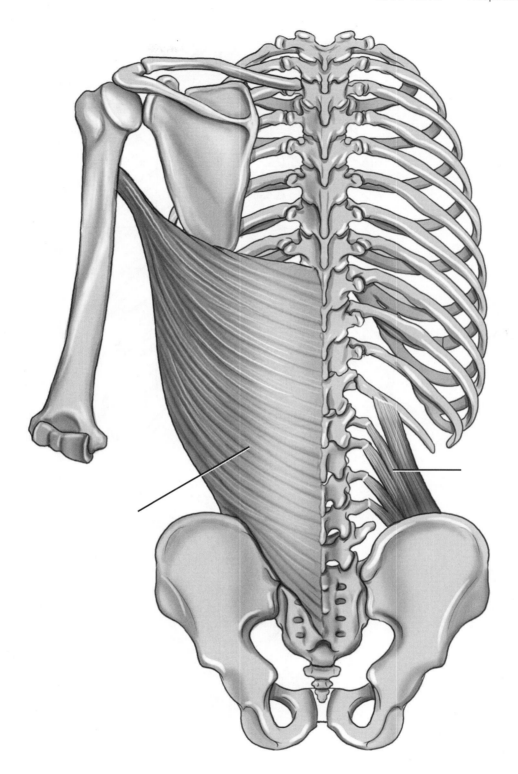

15.

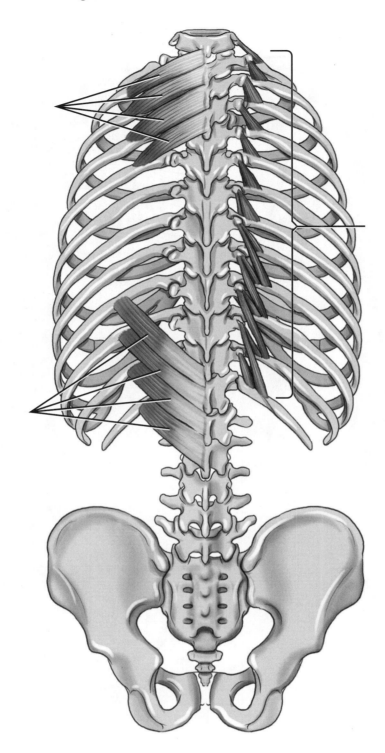

16.

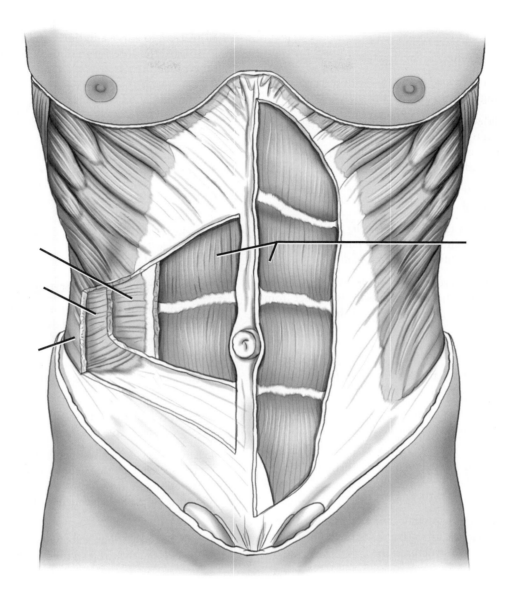

TRUE-FALSE

1. The respiratory tract includes the nasal, oral and pharyngeal cavities, larynx, trachea, and lungs.

2. The lungs are divided into lobes, with three lobes in the left lung and two lobes in the right lung.

3. The ribs attach posteriorly to the corpus and transverse processes of thoracic vertebrae, and for all but two ribs anteriorly to the sternum by means of the ribs' costal cartilages.

4. The vertebrosternal ribs attach to the sternum via a common costal cartilage.

5. Ribs 10, 11, and 12 are called *floating ribs* because they do not attach to the sternum but instead are imbedded in the abdominal musculature.

6. The ribs vary in size, getting progressively larger from ribs 1 through 7 and then progressively smaller from ribs 8 through 12, giving the thoracic framework a barrel-like shape.

FILL IN THE BLANK

1. The ribs that attach to the sternum by means of a common costal cartilage are called _____ ribs.

2. On the pelvis, the ligament that extends from the pubic symphysis to the iliac crest is the _____ ligament.

3. The coxal bone is a paired bone consisting of three lesser bones: the _____, _____, and _____.

4. The pectoral girdle provides the attachment of the upper limbs to the torso (trunk) of the body. It is composed of two structures: the _____ and the _____.

5. The bony skeletal framework for respiration consists of the _____, _____, _____, and _____.

6. An unpaired segmented bone lying in the midline on the superior-anterior thoracic wall that fixes the ventral ends of the ribs' costal cartilages is the _____.

MULTIPLE CHOICE

1. The primary muscles involved in lowering the ribs and sternum and thus participating in the exhalation phase of respiration are located in the _____ region of the body.
   a. thoracic
   b. neck
   c. back
   d. abdominal
   e. all of the above

2. The point on a rib where the rib changes direction, turning to curve anteriorly and then medially toward the anterior midline of the thorax, is called the:
   a. tubercle
   b. head
   c. shaft
   d. neck
   e. none of the above

3. The most posterior portion of the rib that attaches to the corpus of each thoracic vertebra is the:
   a. shaft
   b. neck
   c. head
   d. angle
   e. none of the above

APPLICATION EXERCISES

1. Define and distinguish *intrapulmonary pressure* and *intrathoracic pressure,* and describe their role in the speech production process.

2. Define and distinguish *tidal volume* and *vital capacity* and describe their importance in speech production.

3. Identify each of the types of speech breathing and describe their role in speech production.

4. Discuss the differences between *vegetative breathing* and *speech breathing* in regard to such measures as duration of inhalation vs. exhalation phases, force and control of air, and frequency of respiratory cycles per minute.

5. Define and distinguish between *air pressures* and *airflow* and their role in the speech production process.

6. Identify instrumentation used to study respiratory quantities, including lung volumes, lung capacities, air pressures, and airflow.

7. Describe how the volume of air expended in speech breathing varies with the types of speech sounds produced.

8. What changes in speech breathing occur throughout the lifespan and why? What are the clinical implications of such changes for speech production purposes?

9. What speech breathing problems are associated with the following conditions? Why and how? What are the clinical implications of these speech breathing problems?
   a. Parkinson's disease
   b. cerebral palsy
   c. cervical spinal cord injury

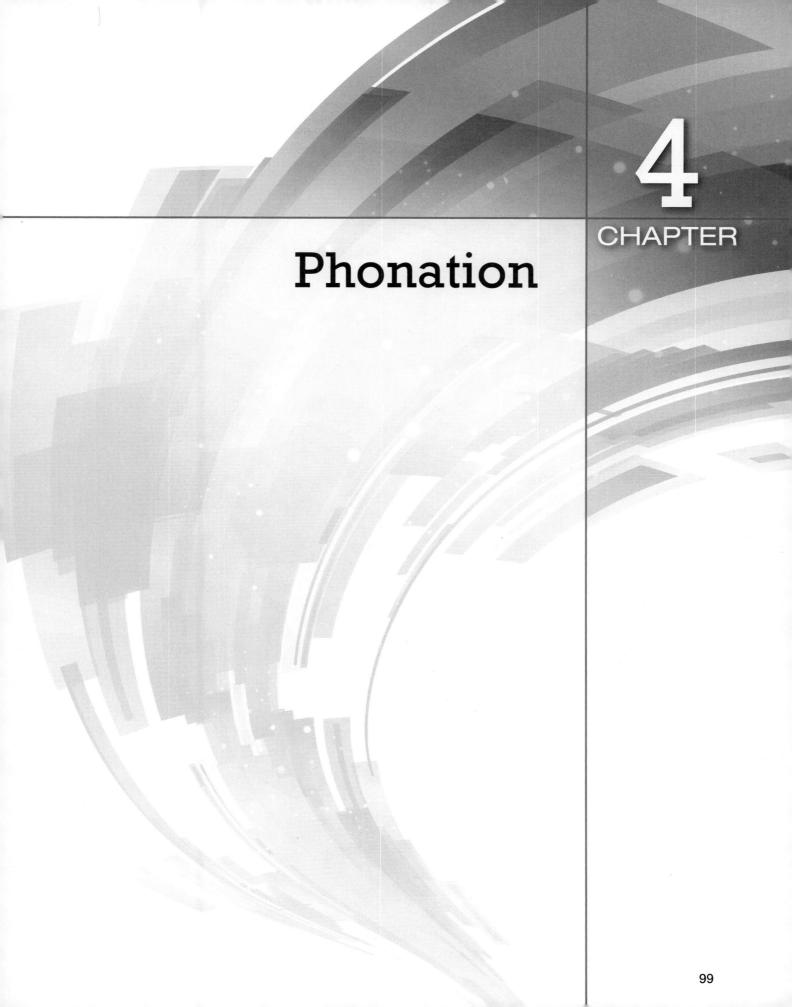

Phonation

CHAPTER 4

THE LARYNX

Phonation, the process of producing voicing (i.e., all voiced speech sounds, including all vowels, diphthongs, and voiced consonants) is controlled by the **larynx**, an unpaired musculo cartilaginous–membranous structure located in the anterior part of the neck. It is connected via ligaments and membranes to the hyoid bone above and the trachea below (Figures 4-1 and 4-2). It provides a smooth, rhythmic pulsation on the air that comes from the lungs, which creates a complex, quasiperiodic signal identified as a speech sound.

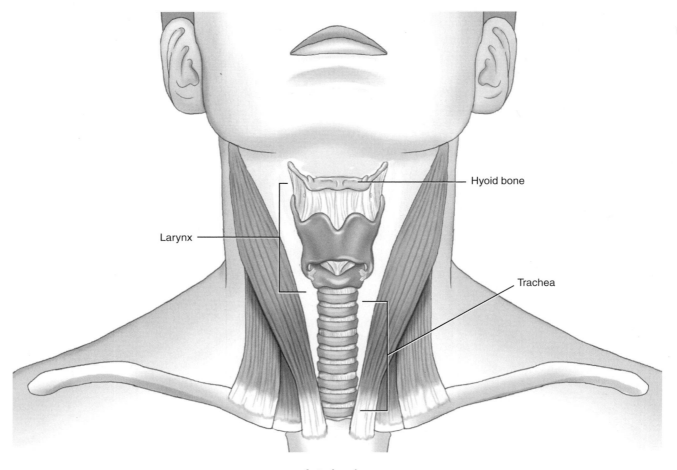

Hyoid bone

Larynx

Trachea

Anterior view

FIGURE 4-1 Location of larynx in neck region.

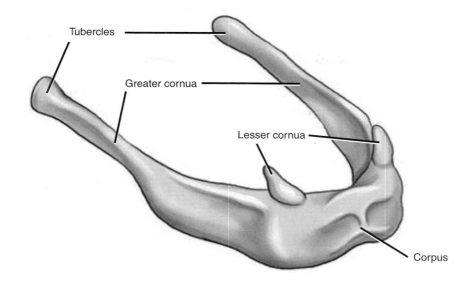

Anterolateral view

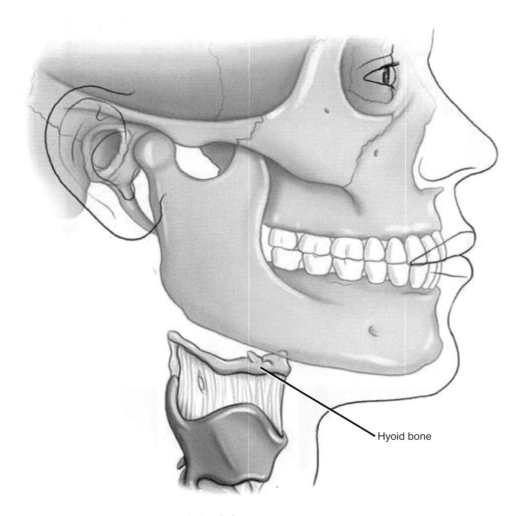

Lateral view

FIGURE 4-2 Hyoid bone and its location in neck region.

SKELETAL FRAMEWORK OF THE LARYNX

The cartilages that compose the skeletal framework of the larynx include three unpaired and three paired cartilages (Figure 4-3). The three unpaired cartilages are the thyroid, cricoid, and epiglottis. The **thyroid cartilage** serves to protect the vocal folds (Figure 4-4). It is the largest of the cartilages and comprises most of the anterior part of the larynx. It is composed of two cartilaginous plates (laminae) fused together; a superior V-shaped thyroid notch at their juncture; an angular protuberance (the Adam's apple); and two sets of "horns," one set projecting upward (superior cornua) and one set projecting downward (inferior cornua).

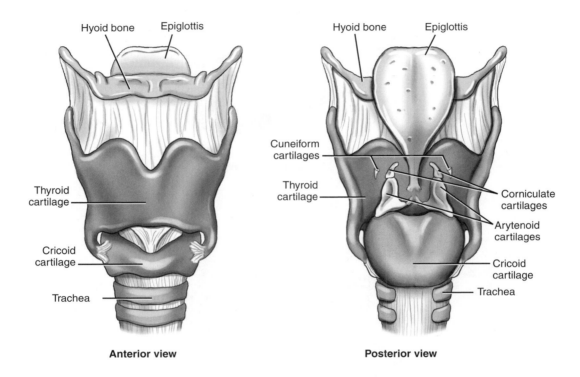

Anterior view

Posterior view

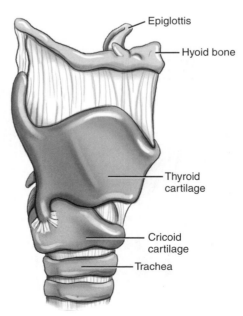

Lateral view

FIGURE 4-3 Cartilages of the larynx.

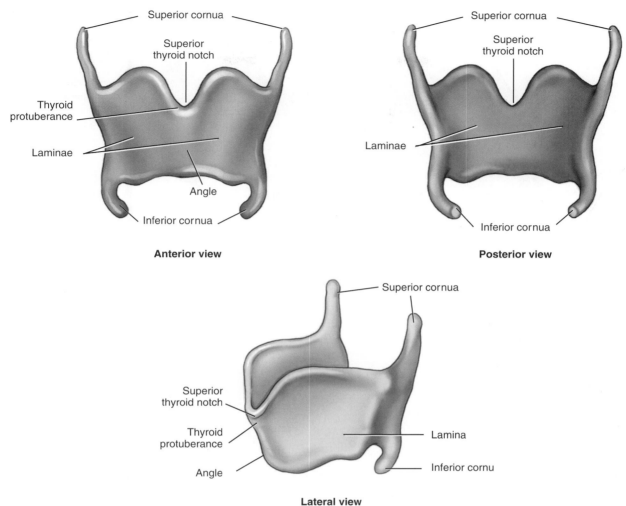

FIGURE 4-4 Thyroid cartilage.

The **cricoid cartilage** is a ring-shaped structure that occupies the most inferior part of the larynx and lies directly above the trachea (Figure 4-5). Its anterior **arch** is narrow, whereas its posterior **quadrate lamina** is large, containing four **articular facets**, two superior and two lateral, for the attachment of the arytenoid cartilages and for articulation with the inferior cornua of the thyroid cartilage, respectively. The posterior **cricoid notch** is a ridge on the midline between the two superior articular facets. The inferior border of the cricoid cartilage attaches to the first ring of the trachea by means of the **cricotracheal membrane**. The **epiglottis** is a leaflike structure behind the hyoid bone and the

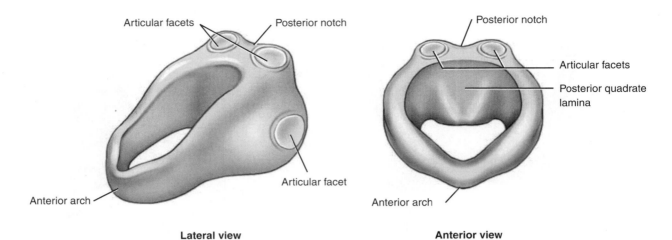

FIGURE 4-5 Cricoid cartilage.

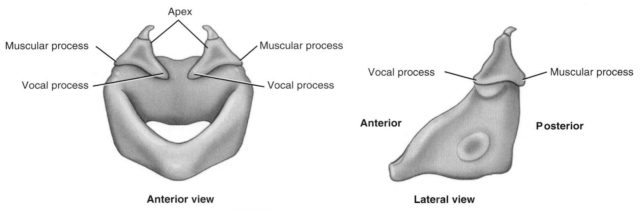

FIGURE 4-6 Arytenoid cartilage.

root of the tongue (Figure 4-3). Its function is to cover the entrance to the larynx during deglutition (swallowing), thereby preventing food or liquid from entering the larynx.

The three paired laryngeal cartilages are the arytenoids, corniculates, and cuneiforms. The pyramid-shaped **arytenoid**

cartilages are located on the sloping posterior border of the cricoid cartilage (Figure 4-6). The **vocal folds** are attached to the arytenoid cartilages and can be approximated in the midline or pulled apart via muscle contraction. The **corniculate cartilages** are located on the top of the apexes of the arytenoid

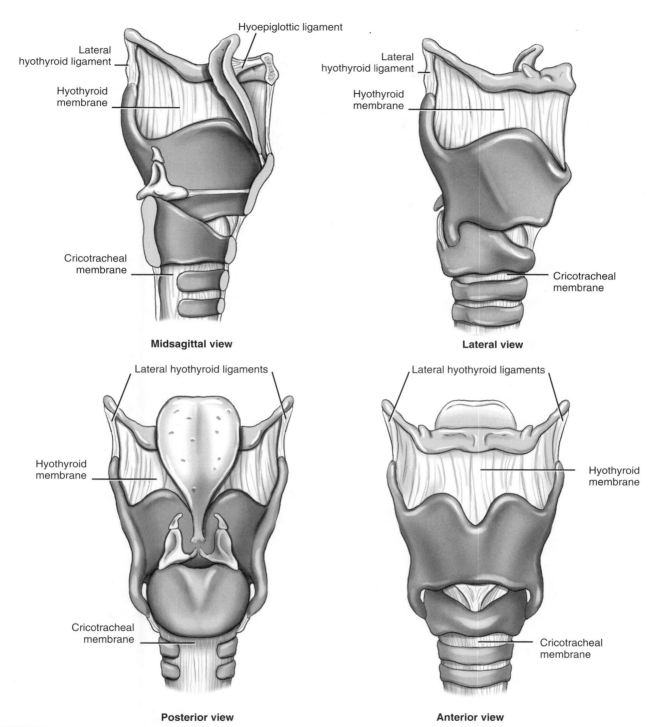

Midsagittal view

Lateral view

Posterior view

Anterior view

FIGURE 4-7 Extrinsic laryngeal membranes: hyothyroid membrane, lateral hyothyroid ligaments, cricotracheal membrane, hyoepiglottic ligament.

cartilages (Figure 4-3). The **cuneiform cartilages**, when present, are embedded in the aryepiglottic folds (Figure 4-3).

The **extrinsic laryngeal membranes** connect the laryngeal cartilages to the structures outside the larynx, either the hyoid bone above or the trachea below (Figure 4-7).

They include the **hyothyroid** (or **thyrohyoid**) **membrane** (connecting the thyroid cartilage to the hyoid bone), **lateral hyothyroid ligaments** (connecting the superior cornua of the thyroid cartilage to the major cornua of the hyoid bone), **hyoepiglottal ligament** (connecting the epiglottis and the hyoid bone), and the **cricotracheal membrane** (connecting the cricoid cartilage and the first ring of the trachea).

The **intrinsic laryngeal membranes** connect the cartilages to each other (Figures 4-8, 4-9, and 4-10). They include the **conus elasticus** (medial cricothyroid ligament and lateral cricothyroid membranes connecting the thyroid, cricoid, and arytenoid cartilages); **quadrangular membranes** (connecting the epiglottis, thyroid, corniculate, and arytenoid cartilages); the **aryepiglottic folds** (extending from the epiglottis to the arytenoid cartilages); the **anterior, lateral,** and **posterior ceratocricoid ligaments** (reinforcing crico-thyroid articulation); the **thyroepiglottic ligament** (attaching the thyroid cartilage to the epiglottis); and the **posterior cricoarytenoid ligament** (attaching the cricoid and arytenoid cartilages).

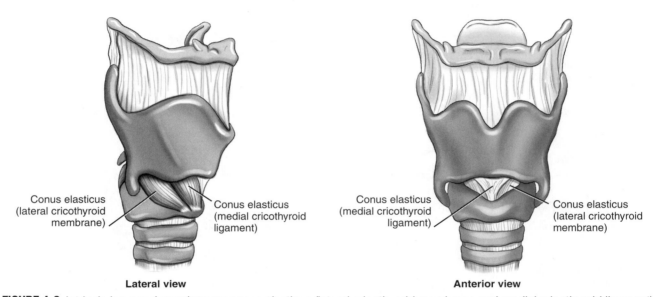

FIGURE 4-8 Intrinsic laryngeal membranes: conus elasticus (lateral cricothyroid membrane and medial cricothyroid ligament).

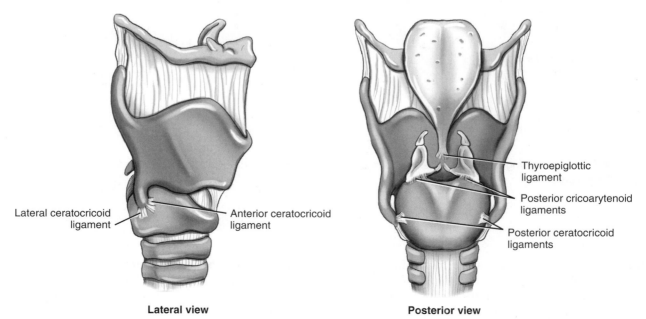

FIGURE 4-9 Intrinsic laryngeal membranes: anterior, lateral, and posterior ceratocricoid ligaments, and thyroepiglottic ligament.

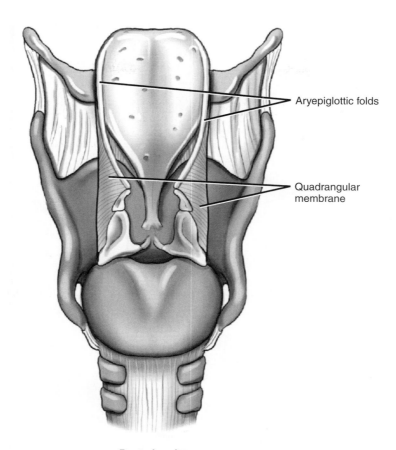

Posterior view

FIGURE 4-10 Intrinsic laryngeal membranes: quadrangular membrane and aryepiglottic folds.

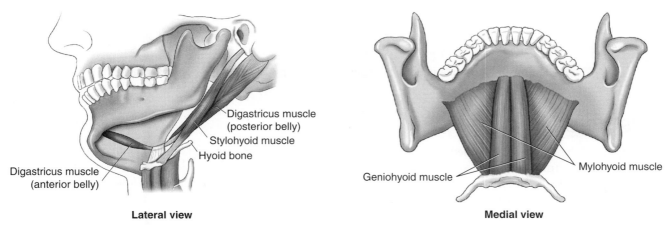

Lateral view   **Medial view**

FIGURE 4-11 Extrinsic supra hyoid laryngeal muscles: digastricus, stylohyoid, mylohyoid, and geniohyoid.

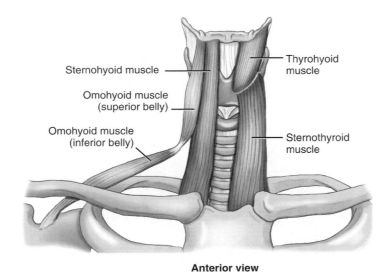

Anterior view

FIGURE 4-12 Extrinsic infra hyoid laryngeal muscles: sternohyoid, omohyoid, thyrohyoid, and sternothyroid.

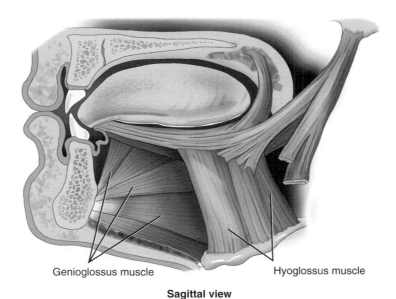

Sagittal view

FIGURE 4-13 Supplementary laryngeal elevators: hyoglossus and genioglossus.

MUSCLES

The muscles of the larynx are classified as either *extrinsic* or *intrinsic*. The extrinsic muscles connect the cartilages to structures outside the larynx, and the intrinsic muscles connect the cartilages to one another.

The **extrinsic laryngeal muscles** are those classified anatomically as lying above (suprahyoid) or below (infrahyoid) the hyoid bone. The **suprahyoid muscles** are the **digastricus**, **stylohyoid**, **mylohyoid**, and **geniohyoid muscles** (Figure 4-11). The **infrahyoid muscles** are the **sternohyoid**, **omohyoid**, **thyrohyoid**, and **sternothyroid** (Figure 4-12). On a functional basis, the extrinsic muscles are classified as *elevators* or *depressors*. The **laryngeal elevators** are all suprahyoid muscles (digastricus, mylohyoid, geniohyoid,

and stylohyoid) and one infrahyoid muscle (thyrohyoid). In addition, there are two muscles of the tongue that are classified as supplementary laryngeal elevators: the **hyoglossus** and **genioglossus** muscles (Figure 4-13). The laryngeal depressors are the other three infrahyoid muscles (sternohyoid, sternothyroid, and omohyoid) (Figure 4-12).

The **intrinsic laryngeal muscles** connect the laryngeal cartilages to each other and are classified according to their function as **vocal-fold abductor** (**posterior cricoarytenoid**), **laryngeal adductors** (**lateral cricoarytenoid**, **transverse arytenoid**, and **oblique arytenoid**), **vocal-fold relaxers** (**lateral cricoarytenoid** and **thyromuscularis**), and **vocal-fold tensors** (**cricothyroid** and **thyrovocalis**) (Figure 4-14).

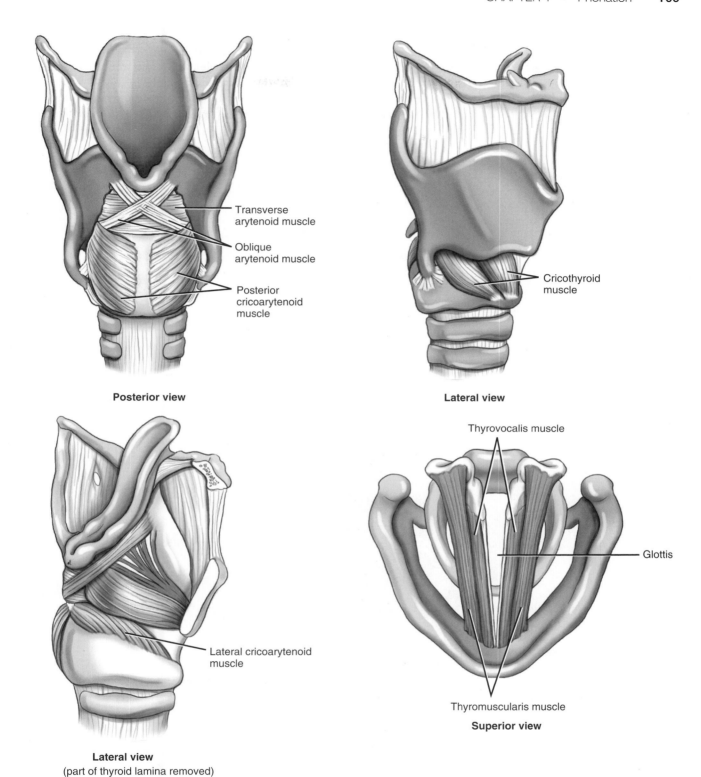

Transverse
arytenoid muscle

Oblique
arytenoid muscle

Posterior
cricoarytenoid
muscle

Cricothyroid
muscle

Posterior view

Lateral view

Thyrovocalis muscle

Glottis

Thyromuscularis muscle

Superior view

Lateral cricoarytenoid
muscle

Lateral view
(part of thyroid lamina removed)

FIGURE 4-14 Intrinsic laryngeal muscles: posterior and lateral cricoarytenoid, transverse and oblique arytenoid, thyromuscularis, thyrovocalis, and cricothyroid.

The variable opening between the vocal folds is called the **glottis**. The width of the glottis is determined by movements of the arytenoid cartilages. Its opening is narrowest during phonation and widest during inhalation. The main mass of the vocal folds is composed of the **thyroarytenoid muscle** (which includes the **thyrovocalis** and **thyromuscularis muscles**. Figure 4-14).

INTERNAL CAVITY

The **internal cavity** (interior) of the larynx as viewed in a frontal sectioning extends from the **aditus laryngis** (laryngeal entrance) above to the inferior border of the cricoid cartilage below (Figure 4-15). It is divided into three main parts: a superior division (the **vestibule**), which extends from the **aditus laryngis** to the **ventricular (false) folds**; the middle division (**ventricle**), which runs from the **ventricular folds** to the true **vocal folds**; and the inferior division (**subglottal region**), which includes the true vocal folds superiorly and the lowest border of the cricoid cartilage inferiorly.

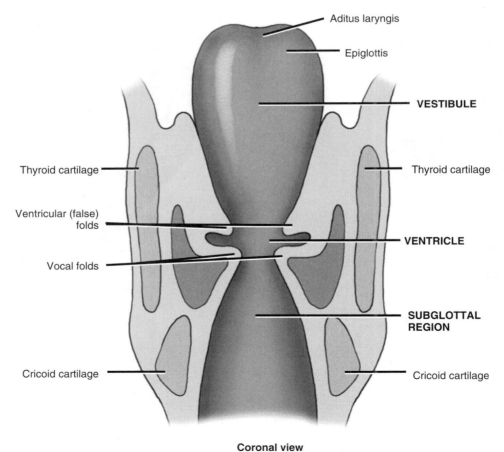

Aditus laryngis

Epiglottis

VESTIBULE

Thyroid cartilage

Thyroid cartilage

Ventricular (false) folds

VENTRICLE

Vocal folds

SUBGLOTTAL REGION

Cricoid cartilage

Cricoid cartilage

Coronal view

FIGURE 4-15 Internal cavity of the larynx.

REVIEW EXERCISES

ANATOMY EXERCISES

LEVEL 1

In the illustrations in Level 1, (a) identify each anatomical structure, and (b) identify each listed part by drawing a line to each part and labeling it.

1. _____

   larynx

   hyoid bone

   trachea

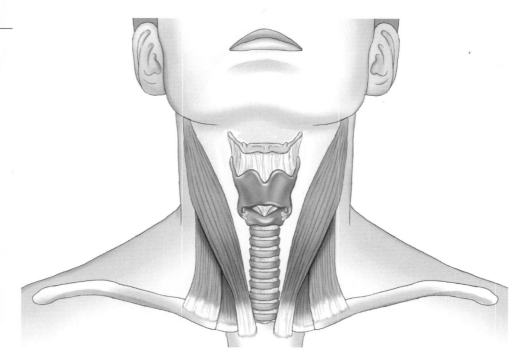

2. _____

    corpus

    tubercles

    greater cornua

    lesser cornua

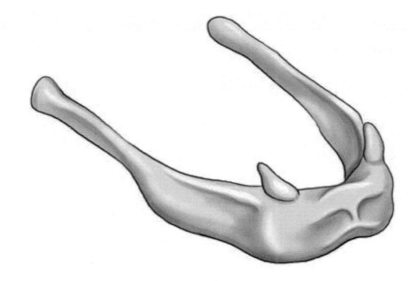

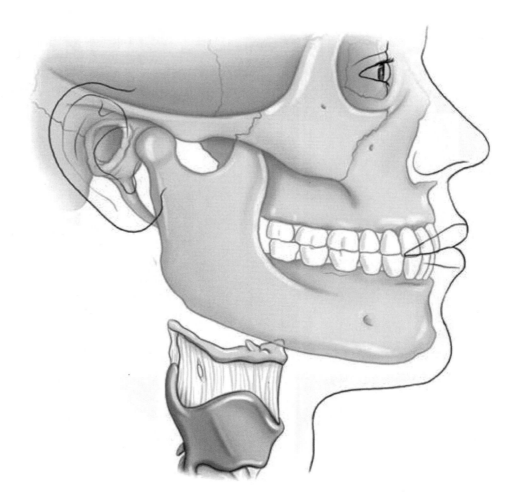

3. _____

thyroid

cricoid

epiglottis

arytenoid

corniculate

cuneiform

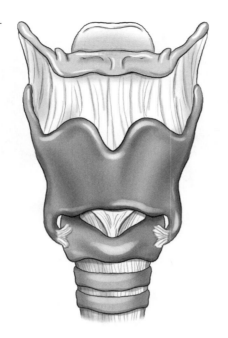 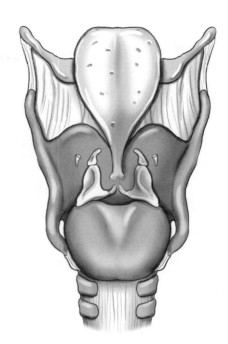

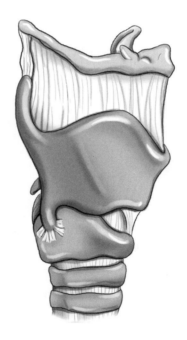

4. _____

laminae

angle

protuberance

superior cornua

inferior cornua

superior notch

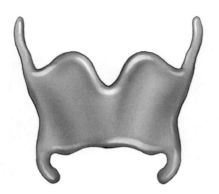
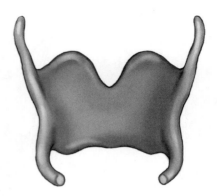
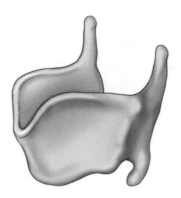

5. _____

anterior arch

posterior quadrate
lamina

articular facets

posterior notch

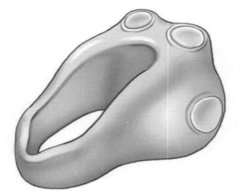 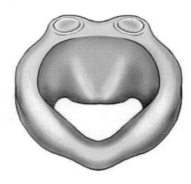

6. _____

apex

muscular processes

vocal processes

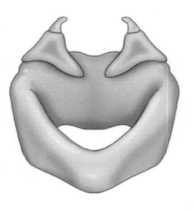 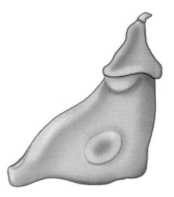

7. _____

   hyothyroid membrane

   lateral hyothyroid
   ligaments

   hyoepiglottic ligament

   cricotracheal
   membrane

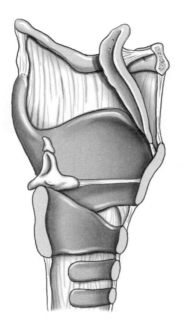

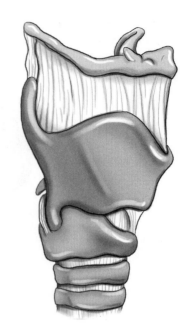

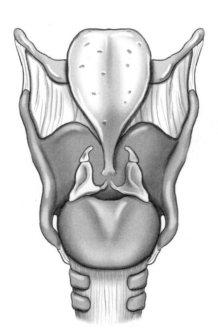

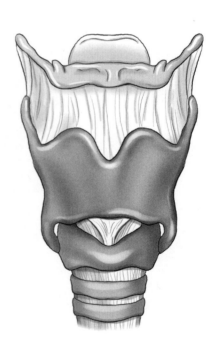

8. _____

medial cricothyroid
ligament

lateral cricothyroid
membranes

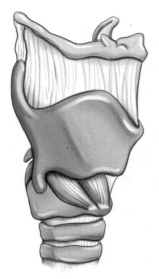
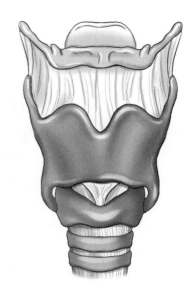

9. _____

anterior ceratocricoid
ligament

posterior ceratocricoid
ligament

lateral ceratocricoid
ligament

thyroepiglottic
ligament

posterior
cricoarytenoid
ligaments

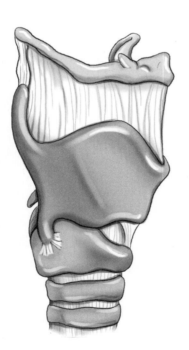
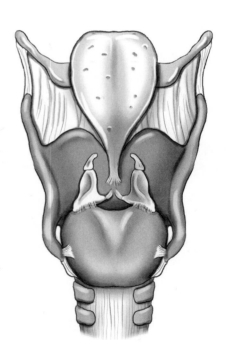

10. _____

quadrangular
membrane

aryepiglottic folds

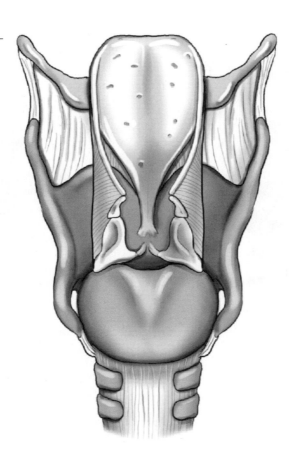

11. _____

digastricus muscle
(anterior belly)

digastricus muscle
(posterior belly)

stylohyoid muscle

mylohyoid muscle

geniohyoid muscle

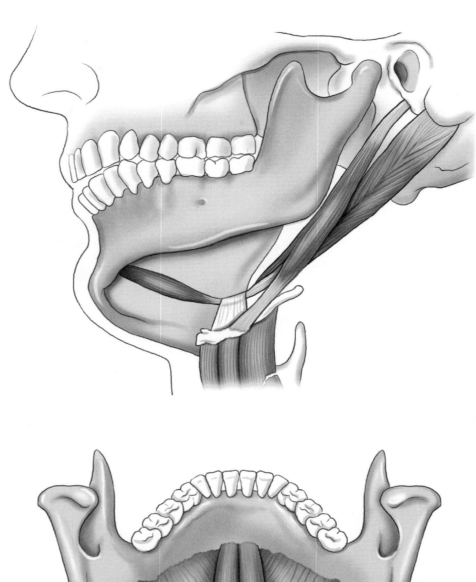

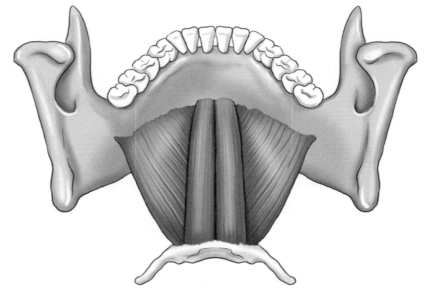

12. _____

   sternohyoid muscle

   omohyoid muscle
   (superior belly)

   omohyoid muscle
   (inferior belly)

   thyrohyoid muscle

   sternothyroid muscle

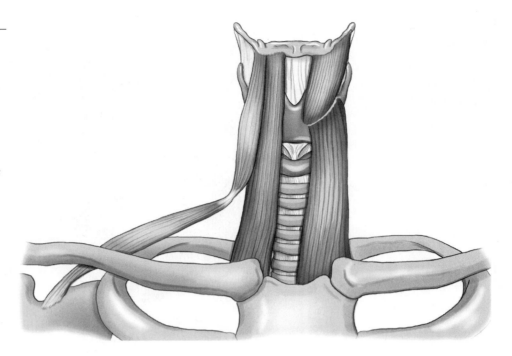

13. _____

genioglossus muscle

hypoglossus muscle

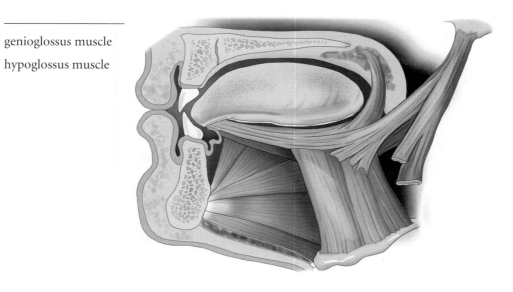

14. _____

posterior
cricoarytenoid

lateral cricoarytenoid

oblique arytenoid

transverse arytenoid

thyrovocalis

thyromuscularis

cricothyroid

glottis

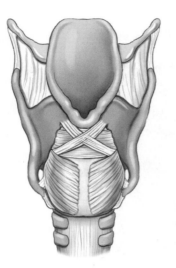
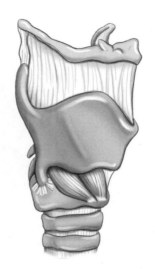
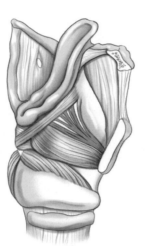
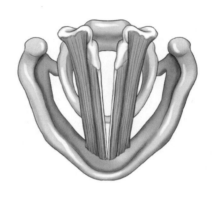

15. _____

    vestibule

    ventricle

    subglottal region

    aditus laryngis

    ventricular (false)
    vocal folds

    true vocal folds

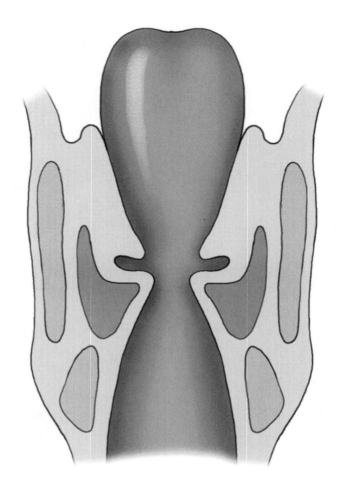

LEVEL 2

In Level 2, identify each anatomical part indicated by lines in the illustrations below.

  1.

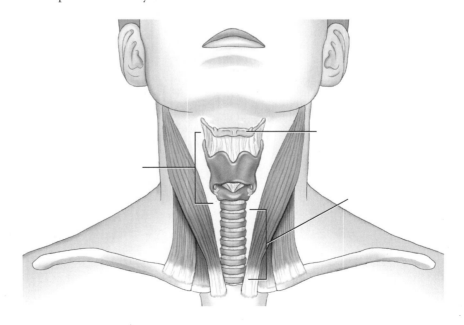

2.

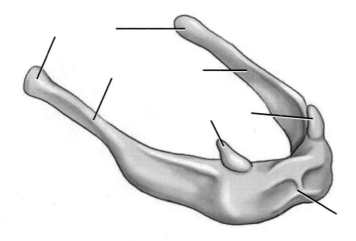

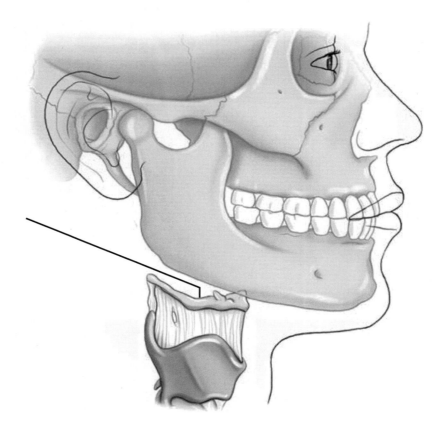

3.

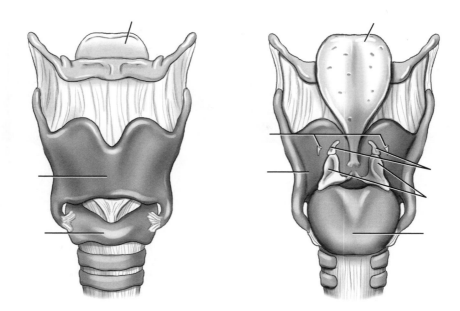

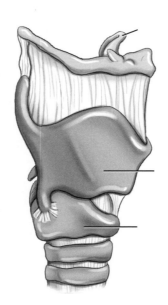

4.

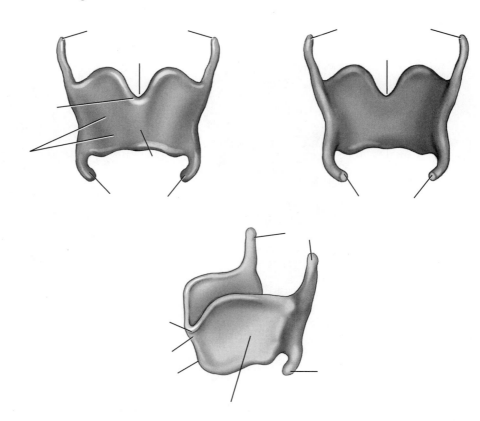

5.

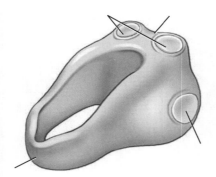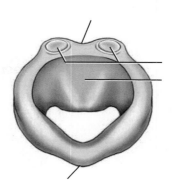

6.

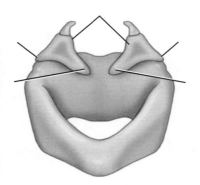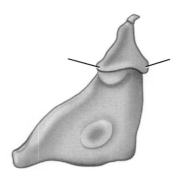

7.

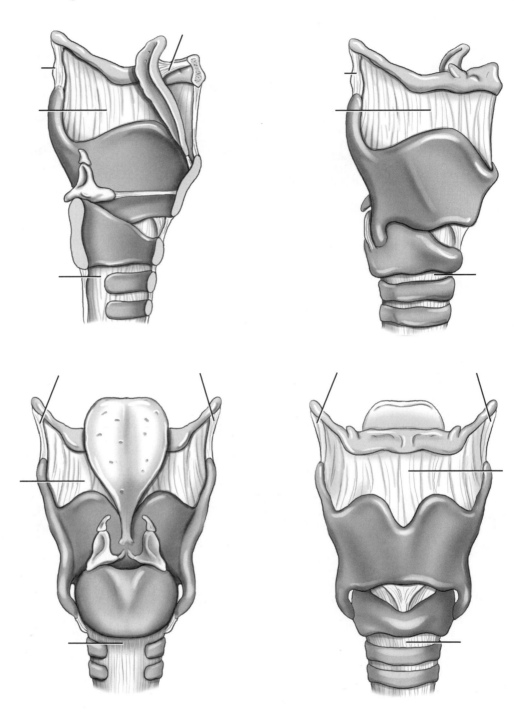

8.

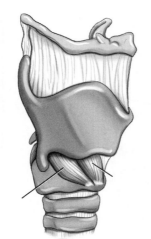 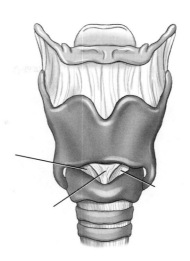

9.

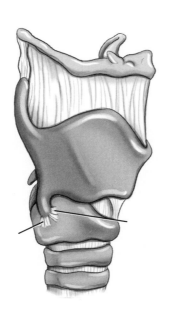 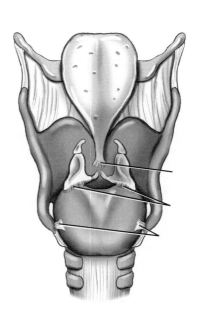

10.

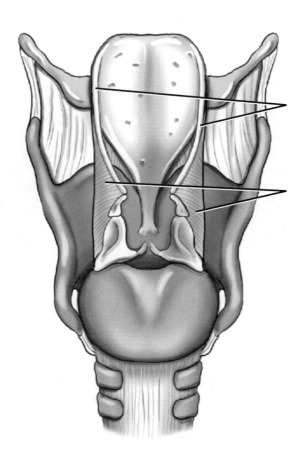

11.

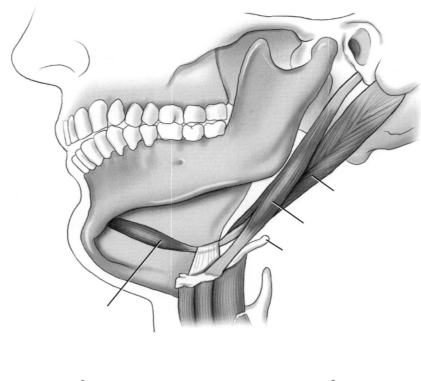

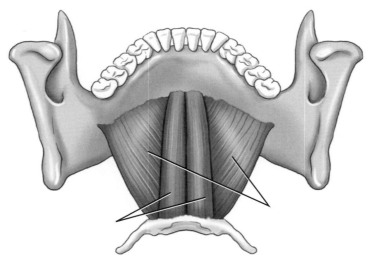

12.

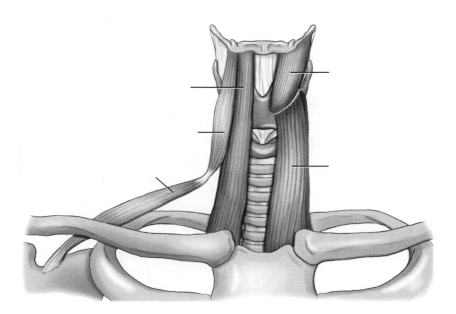

13.

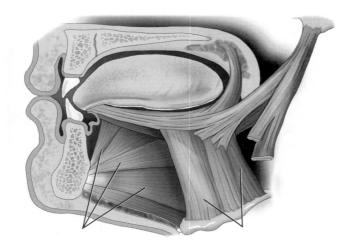

14.

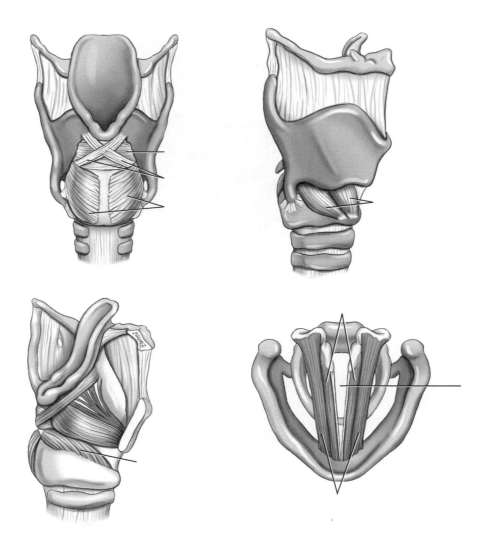

15.

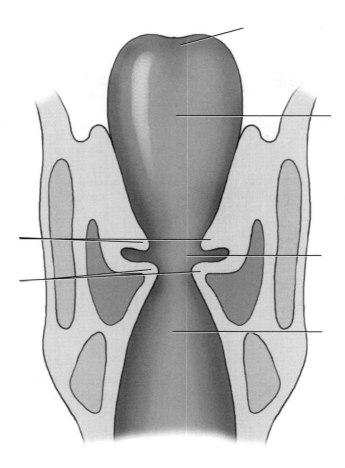

TRUE-FALSE

1. The process of phonation is involved in the production of all vowels, diphthongs, and consonants.

2. Paired laryngeal cartilages include the arytenoid, epiglottis, and corniculate.

3. Extrinsic laryngeal membranes connect the cartilages of the larynx to the hyoid bone above or the trachea below.

4. Extrinsic laryngeal muscles are classified anatomically as laryngeal elevators and laryngeal depressors.

5. The lateral border of the vocal folds is attached to the thyroid cartilage, while the medial border of the vocal folds is free, unattached to any cartilage.

6. The opening of the glottis is widest during inhalation and narrowest during phonation.

7. Unpaired laryngeal cartilages include the thyroid, corniculate, and cricoid.

8. The superior division of the internal cavity of the larynx extends from the aditus laryngis to the true vocal folds.

9. Infrahyoid muscles of the larynx include the digastricus, mylohyoid, geniohyoid, and stylohyoid muscles.

FILL IN THE BLANK

1. The space between the vocal folds when they are in an abducted position is called the _____.

2. When the lateral cricoarytenoid muscle contracts, the _____ cartilages are pulled forward, thereby approximating their anterior portions in the midline, which approximates the _____ in the midline.

3. The free, unattached upper margin of the vocal folds is called the _____.

4. The contraction of the _____, _____, and _____ muscles is necessary to achieve

approximation of the vocal folds in the appropriate adducted position to be set into vibration.

5. The laryngeal cartilages, located on top of the posterior quadrate lamina of the cricoid cartilage, are the _____ cartilages.

6. An unpaired cartilage of the larynx that is shaped like a signet ring and forms the lower portion of the larynx is the _____ cartilage.

7. A paired laryngeal ligament that extends from the superior cornua of the thyroid cartilage to the greater cornua of the hyoid bone is the _____ ligament.

8. The cricoid cartilage's posterior quadrate lamina contains two superior articular facets for the attachment of the _____ cartilages.

9. The largest of the laryngeal cartilages that forms most of the anterior and lateral walls of the larynx is the _____ cartilage.

10. A bone in the neck region from which the larynx is somewhat suspended is the _____ bone.

11. The internal cavity of the larynx is divided into three main portions: _____, _____, and _____.

MULTIPLE CHOICE

1. Extrinsic laryngeal membranes include the:
   a. conus elasticus
   b. thyroepiglottic ligament
   c. lateral hyothyroid ligaments
   d. all of the above
   e. none of the above

2. Suprahyoid muscles of the larynx include the:
   a. omohyoid
   b. thyrohyoid
   c. stylohyoid
   d. all of the above
   e. none of the above

3. The middle division of the internal cavity of the larynx that extends from the false folds to the true vocal folds, is the:
   a. vestibule
   b. aditus laryngis
   c. subglottis
   d. ventricle
   e. none of the above

4. The vocal fold adductor muscles of the larynx include the:
   a. oblique arytenoid
   b. lateral cricoarytenoid
   c. transverse arytenoid
   d. all of the above
   e. none of the above

5. The vocal fold tensor muscles of the larynx include the:
   a. cricothyroid
   b. ceratocricoid
   c. thyroepiglottic
   d. all of the above
   e. none of the above

6. Extrinsic laryngeal muscle(s) of the larynx include the:
   a. lateral cricoarytenoid
   b. cricothyroid
   c. thyromuscularis
   d. all of the above
   e. none of the above

7. The abductor muscle(s) of the vocal folds is(are) the:
   a. lateral cricoarytenoid
   b. cricothyroid
   c. thyromuscularis
   d. all of the above
   e. none of the above

APPLICATION EXERCISES

1. Define *jitter* and *shimmer,* describe how they are measured, and discuss the clinical application of these vocal measures in the diagnosis and treatment of communication disorders.

2. Define *vocal fundamental frequency* and describe its physiological, acoustical, and perceptual determinants. What is considered the normal range of vocal fundamental frequency for children, adult females, and adult males?

3. Describe how the voice changes with age, including the effect of aging on various physiological, acoustical, and perceptual characteristics of the voice.

4. Describe vocal fold motion, including the phases of vocal fold vibration as well as the cartilaginous and muscular interactions in adduction and abduction of the folds.

Articulation

The skeletal framework for the articulatory process involves the bones of the skull, which are divided into two major parts: the **cranium** (which protects the brain) and the **facial skeleton** (which forms the structural framework for most of the articulators). The facial bones include the mandible, maxillae, nasal, palatine, lacrimal, zygomatic, inferior nasal conchae, and vomer bones (Figures 5-1, 5-2, and 5-3). The cranial bones include the frontal, occipital, ethmoid, sphenoid, parietal, and temporal bones.

The articulatory process involves numerous structures within the oral, nasal, and pharyngeal cavities (Figure 5-4). These are the articulators, which include the lips, tongue, teeth, alveolar ridge, hard palate, and soft palate.

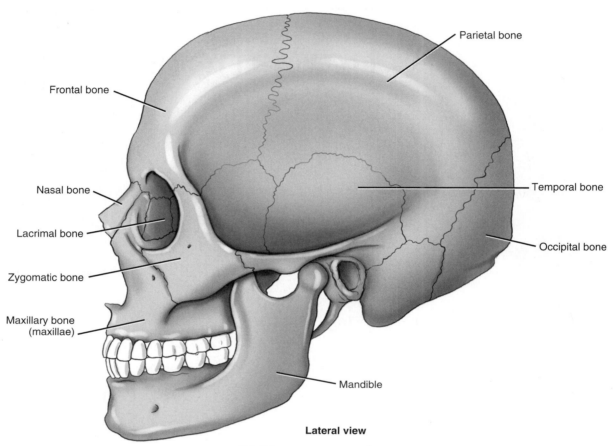

Lateral view

FIGURE 5-1 Facial bones.

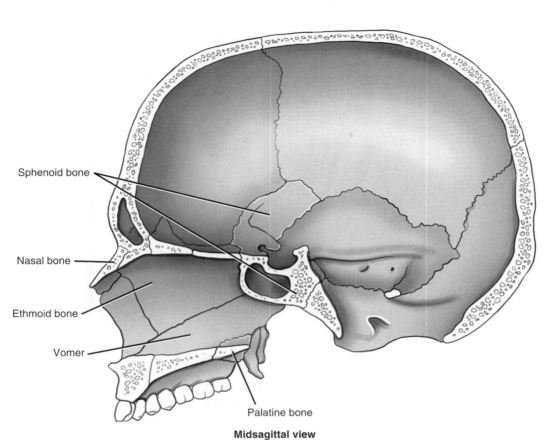

Midsagittal view

FIGURE 5-2 Facial bones.

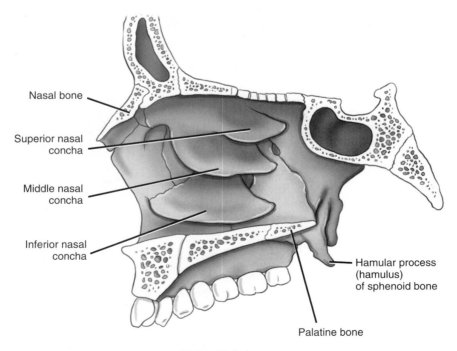

Midsagittal view

FIGURE 5-3 Facial bones.

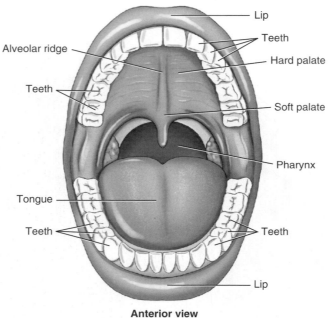

Anterior view

FIGURE 5-4 Oral cavity.

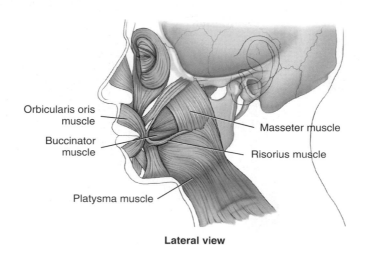

Lateral view

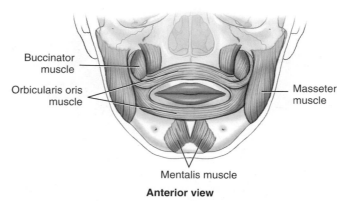

Anterior view

FIGURE 5-5 Muscles of the face and lips.

LIPS AND FACE

The **lips**, which are covered externally by skin and internally by mucous membrane, form the opening of the oral cavity. The muscles of the lips and face provide the lip's mobility. The major lip muscle is the **orbicularis oris**, which completely encircles the mouth. It contains muscle fibers

exclusive to the lips as well as muscle fibers from other muscles of the face that insert into the lips. In addition to their function in facial expression, the muscles of the face and lips also function in the production of speech sounds. Examples of these muscles are the **buccinator**, **risorius**, **mentalis**, and **platysma** (Figure 5-5).

TONGUE

The primary articulator, which is responsible for the production of all English vowels and many consonants, is the tongue. The tongue is a large muscle that composes the floor of the oral cavity (Figure 5-6). Its most anterior portion is the tip, which is very important for producing numerous sounds in English (e.g., /t/, /d/, /s/, /n/, and /l/). The tongue is a mobile structure capable of different movements in the oral cavity. Oral and pharyngeal cavity shapes depend on the position of the various tongue parts at any point in time. Furthermore, the tip of the tongue can move independently of the remainder of the tongue so that the tongue can coarticulate with itself, thereby allowing for the simultaneous movement of different tongue parts to produce different speech sounds.

The muscles of the tongue provide its extensive mobility. They include extrinsic muscles (**genioglossus**, **styloglossus**, **palatoglossus**, and **hyoglossus**) (Figure 5-7) and intrinsic muscles (**superior longitudinal**, **inferior longitudinal**, **transverse**, and **vertical**) (Figure 5-8).

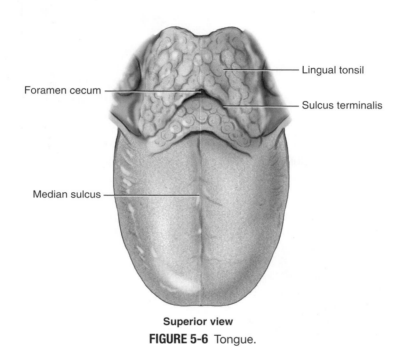

Superior view

FIGURE 5-6 Tongue.

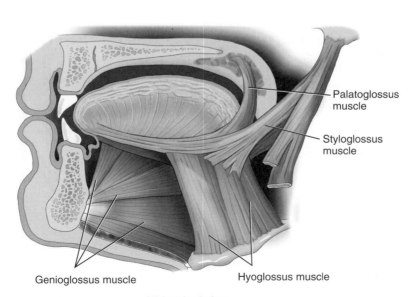

Midsagittal view

FIGURE 5-7 Extrinsic muscles of the tongue.

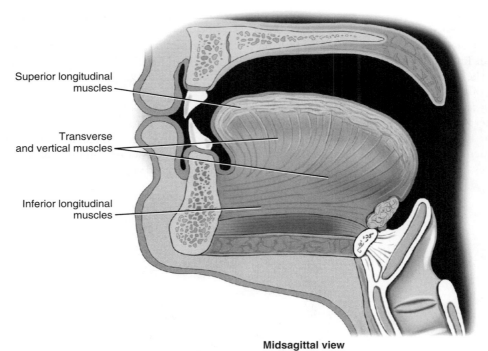

Superior longitudinal
muscles

Transverse
and vertical muscles

Inferior longitudinal
muscles

Midsagittal view

FIGURE 5-8 Intrinsic muscles of the tongue.

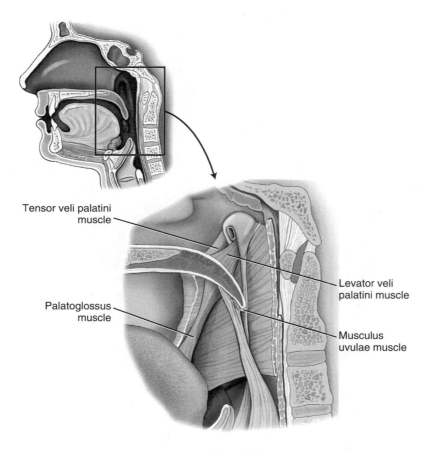

Tensor veli palatini
muscle

Palatoglossus
muscle

Levator veli
palatini muscle

Musculus
uvulae muscle

Midsagittal view

FIGURE 5-9 Muscles of the soft palate.

PALATE

The **soft palate (velum)**, muscular soft tissue in the posterior portion of the hard palate, is attached anteriorly to the free posterior border of the palatine bone. Because the velum can be raised, lowered, or tensed, it may modify the resonance of the vocal tract. The soft palate is lowered (in a relaxed position) for the three nasal sounds of English (/m/, /n/, and /ŋ/) and raised for all other (oral) sounds by making contact with the posterior pharyngeal wall. It thereby achieves velopharyngeal closure by separating the nasal cavity from the oral and pharyngeal cavities. The muscles of the soft palate include the **levator veli palatini**, **musculus uvulae**, **glossopalatinus (palatoglossus)**, **pharyngopalatinus (palatopharyngeus)**, and **tensor veli palatini** (Figure 5-9).

The **alveolar (gum) ridge** lies just behind the upper central incisors and serves as an important contact point in the production of tongue-tip sounds (e.g., /t/, /d/, /s/, /l/, and /n/) (Figure 5-4).

The **hard palate** is composed of the two palatine processes of the maxillae (Figure 5-10). Each palatine process articulates with the palatine process from the other side to form the anterior three fourths of the bony roof of the mouth and the floor of the nasal cavity, thus providing a divider between the two cavities. The hard palate is covered by mucous membrane and **rugae**, small ridges and wrinkles. The **median raphe** is a ridge that lies posterior to the rugae and runs posteriorly in a median line throughout the entire hard palate. It is a contact point for linguapalatal consonants (/ʃ/ and /ʒ/).

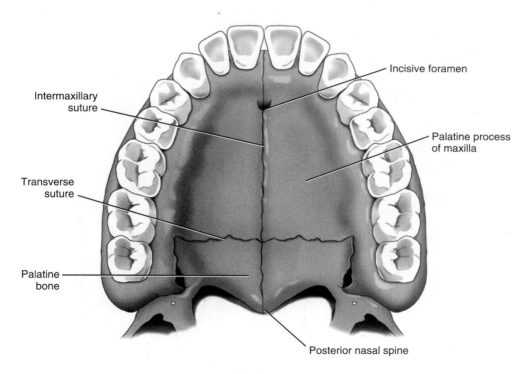

Labels: Intermaxillary suture, Transverse suture, Palatine bone, Incisive foramen, Palatine process of maxilla, Posterior nasal spine

Inferior view

FIGURE 5-10 Hard palate.

PHARYNX

The **pharynx** serves for speech production purposes as a link between the oral cavity, nasal cavity, and larynx (Figure 5-11). It is subdivided into the **nasopharynx**, **oropharynx**, and **laryngopharynx**. In addition, the pharynx is not only a contact point for the posterior portion of the tongue during articulation, but also serves as an important part of the velopharyngeal port mechanism, which is crucial for regulating nasal cavity activity during speech sound production. The pharynx connects the nasal cavity to the auditory tube of the middle ear, thereby equalizing atmospheric and middle ear cavity pressures. The muscles responsible for pharyngeal movement include three **constrictor muscles** (**inferior**, **middle**, and **superior**) as well as the **stylopharyngeus** and **salpingopharyngeus** (Figure 5-12).

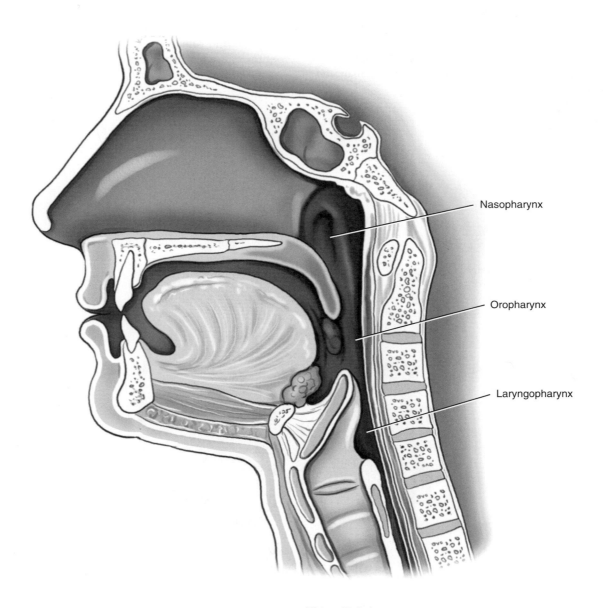

Nasopharynx

Oropharynx

Laryngopharynx

Midsagittal view

FIGURE 5-11 Pharyngeal cavity.

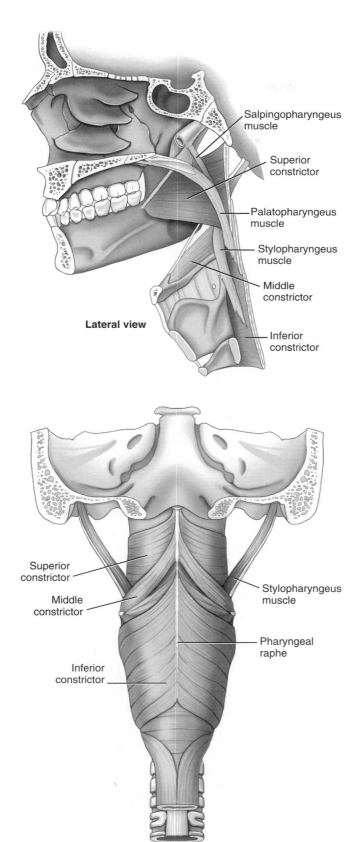

Lateral view

Salpingopharyngeus muscle

Superior constrictor

Palatopharyngeus muscle

Stylopharyngeus muscle

Middle constrictor

Inferior constrictor

Superior constrictor

Middle constrictor

Inferior constrictor

Stylopharyngeus muscle

Pharyngeal raphe

Posterior view

FIGURE 5-12 Muscles of the pharynx.

MANDIBLE

The **mandible** is the largest facial bone, forming the lower jaw (Figure 5-13). It consists of a curved, horizontal portion, the **corpus**; the midline juncture of the two sides of the corpus (**mental symphysis**); and two perpendicular portions, the **rami**, which unite with the ends of the corpus nearly at right angles. There are four processes at the superior portion of the rami, two anterior processes (the **coronoid processes**) and two posterior processes (the **condyloid processes** [or **condyles**]).

The muscles of the mandible are responsible for its movement in speech production as well as for opening, closing, and grinding action. On a functional basis, they are classified as *mandibular depressors* and *mandibular elevators*

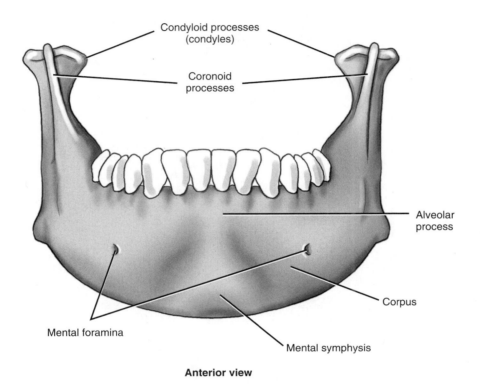

Anterior view

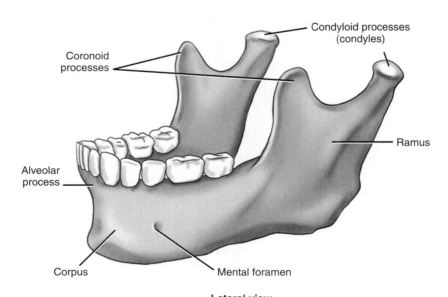

Lateral view

FIGURE 5-13 Mandible.

(Figure 5-14). Mandibular depressors include the **digastricus**, **mylohyoid**, **geniohyoid**, and **lateral pterygoid** muscles. Mandibular elevators include the **masseter**, **temporalis**, and **medial pterygoid** muscles. The sole mandibular protractor muscle is the **lateral (external) pterygoid** muscle. In addition to its primary biological function in mastication (chewing), the mandible contributes to speech production by modifying the resonant characteristics of the oral cavity. The necessary mobility of the mandible requires a normal **temporomandibular joint**, the connection of the mandible to the temporal bone of the skull via ligaments.

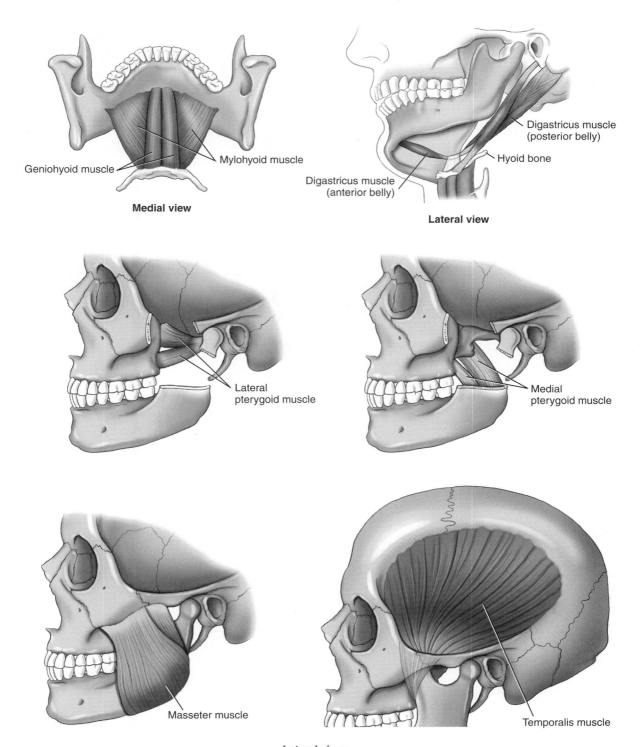

FIGURE 5-14 Muscles of the mandible.

REVIEW EXERCISES

ANATOMY EXERCISES

LEVEL 1

In the illustrations in Level 1, (a) identify each anomical structure, and (b) identify each listed part by drawing a line to each part and labeling it.

1. _____

    frontal bone

    parietal bone

    occipital bone

    temporal bone

    nasal bone

    lacrimal bone

    zygomatic bone

    maxillary bone
    (maxillae)

    mandible

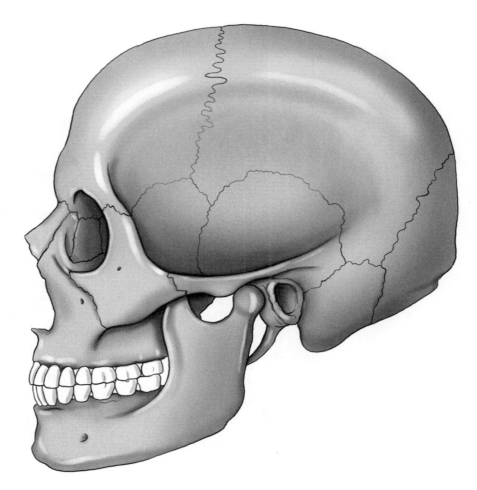

2. _____

    sphenoid bone

    ethmoid bone

    vomer

    nasal bone

    palatine bone

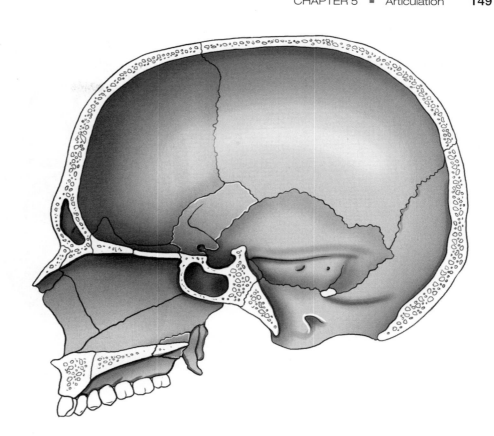

3. _____

    nasal bone

    palatine bone

    inferior nasal conchae

    middle nasal concha

    superior nasal concha

    sphenoid bone (hamular process)

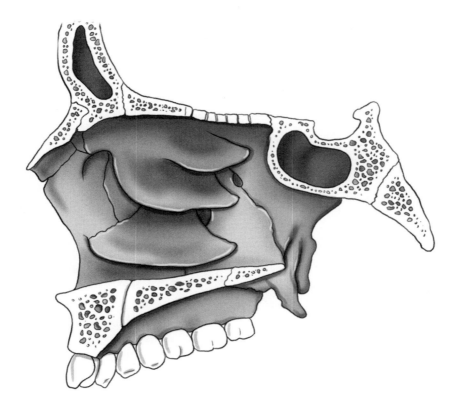

4. _____

    tongue

    lips

    teeth

    alveolar ridge

    hard palate

    soft palate

    pharynx

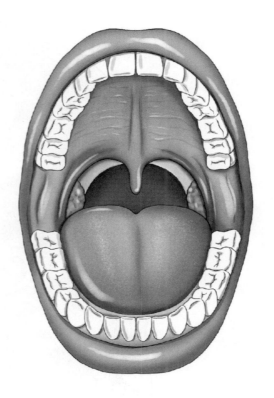

5. _____

buccinator muscle

risorius muscle

mentalis muscle

platysma muscle

orbicularis oris muscle

masseter muscle

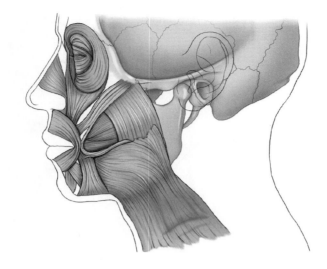

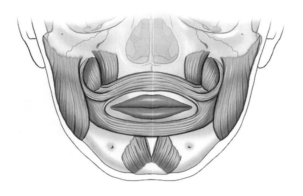

6. _____

median sulcus

sulcus terminalis

foramen cecum

lingual tonsil

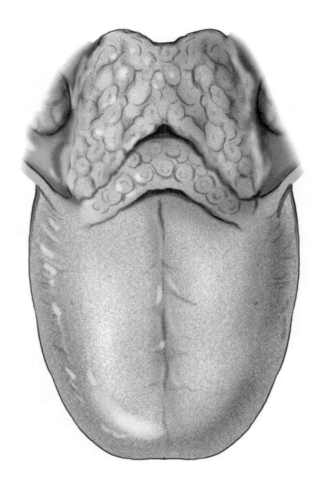

7. _____

genioglossus muscle

styloglossus muscle

palatoglossus muscle

hyoglossus muscle

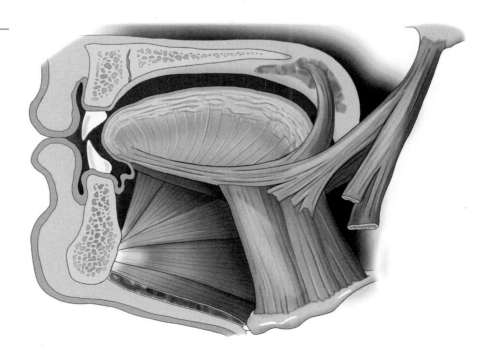

8. _____

superior longitudinal
muscle

inferior longitudinal
muscle

transverse and vertical
muscles

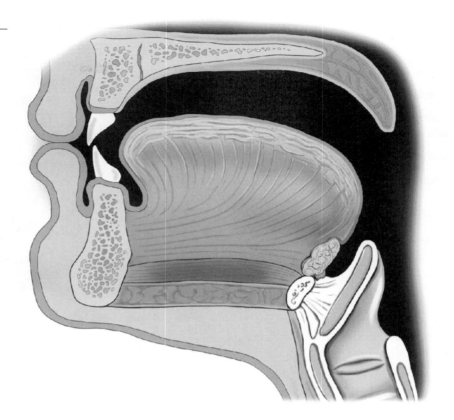

9. _____

levator veli palatini
muscle

tensor veli palatini
muscle

musculus uvulae

palatoglossus muscle

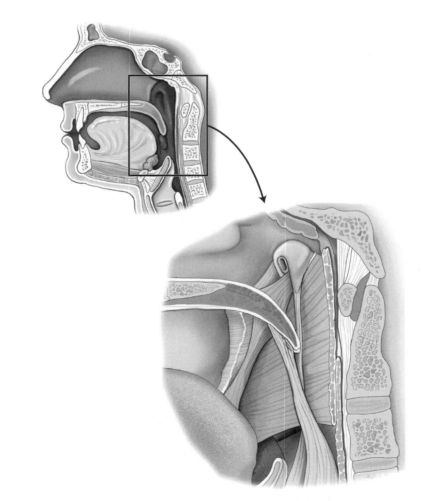

10. _____

    intermaxillary suture

    transverse suture

    incisive foramen

    palatine process of
    maxilla

    posterior nasal spine

    palantine bone

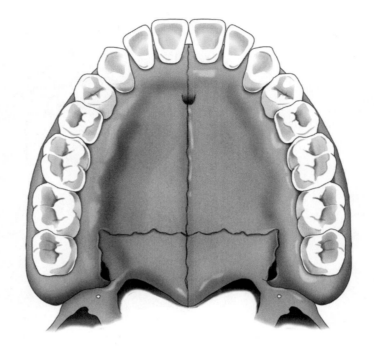

11. _____

nasopharynx

oropharynx

laryngopharynx

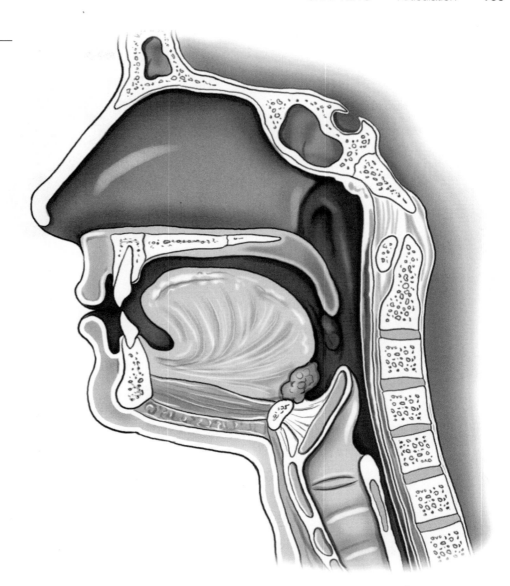

12. _____

inferior constrictor

middle constrictor

superior constrictor

stylopharyngeus

salpingopharyngeus

palatopharyngeus

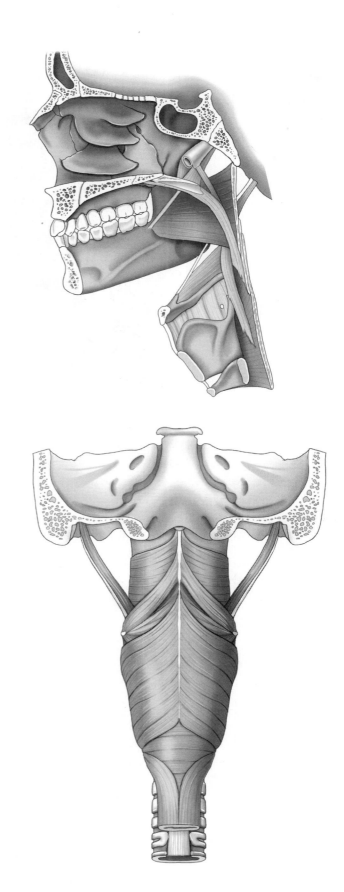

13. _____

corpus

alveolar process

mental foramina

mental symphysis

ramus

coronoid processes

condyloid processes
(condyles)

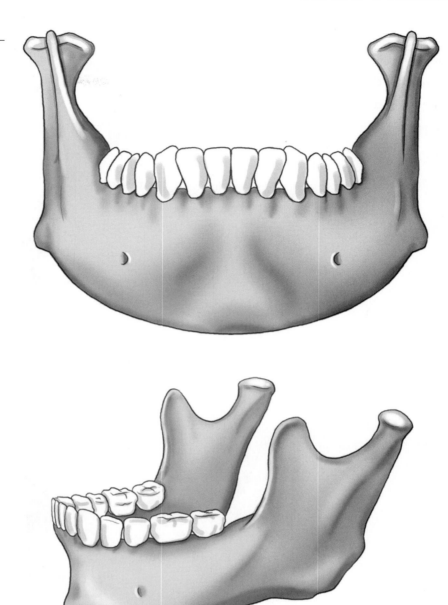

14. _____

masseter muscle

temporalis muscle

medial pterygoid muscle

lateral pterygoid muscle

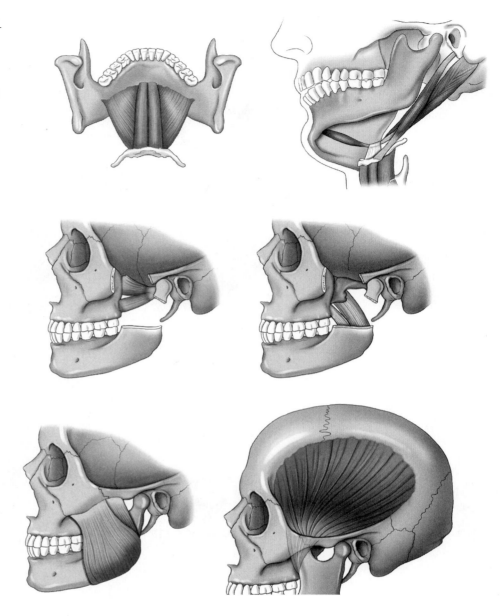

LEVEL 2

In Level 2, identify each anatomical part indicated by lines in the illustrations below.

1.

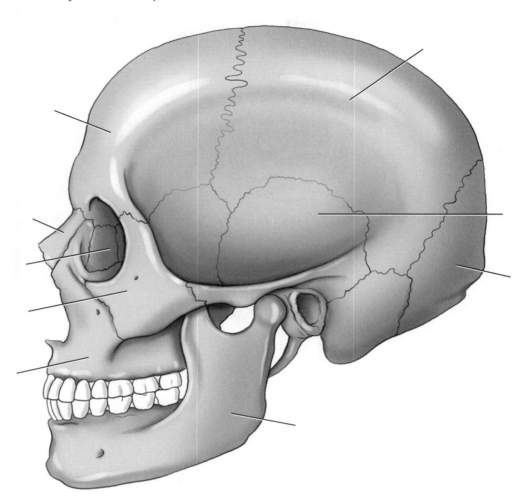

2.

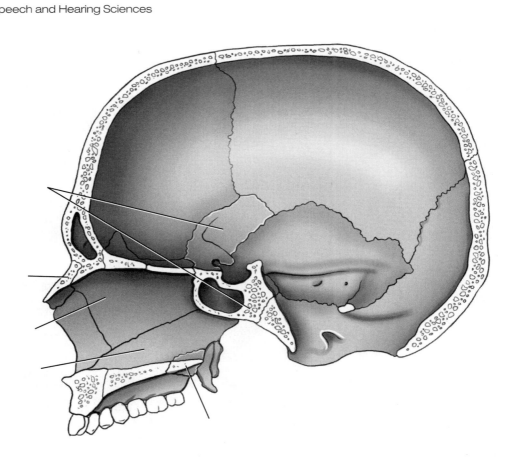

3.

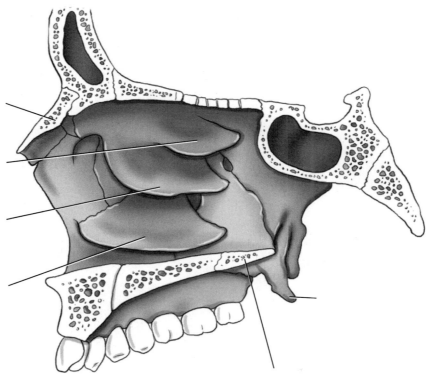

4.

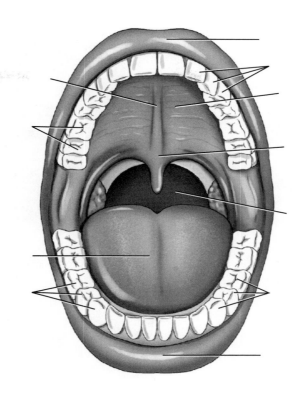

5.

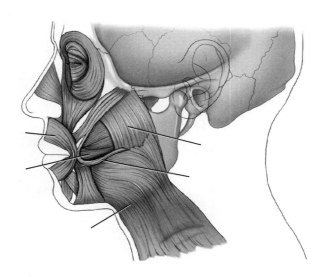

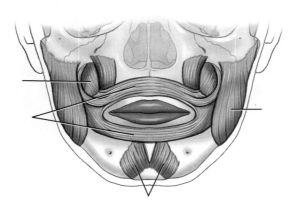

6.

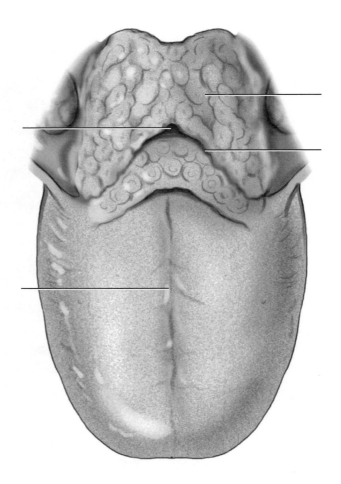

7.

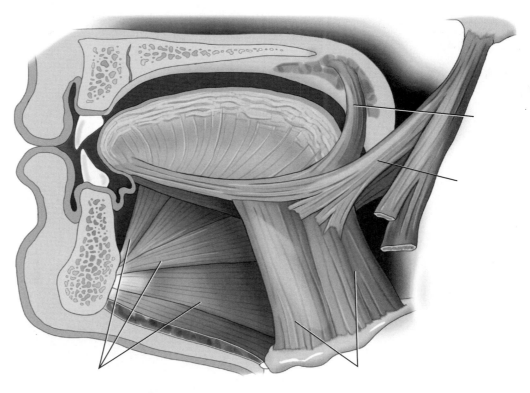

8.

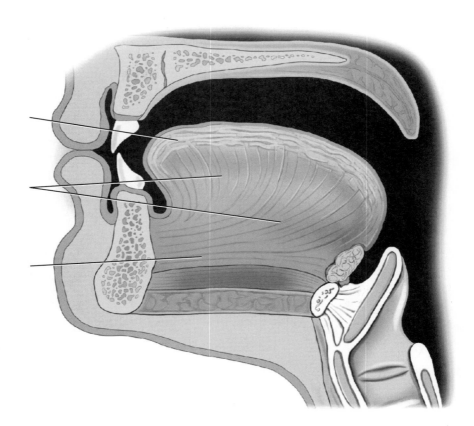

9.

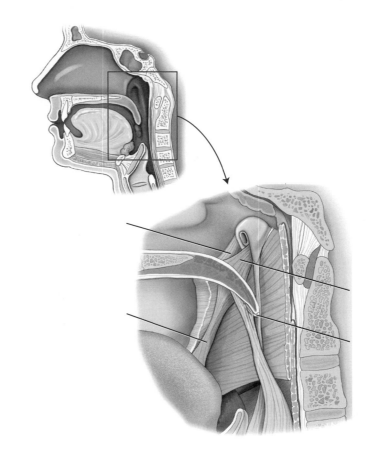

10.

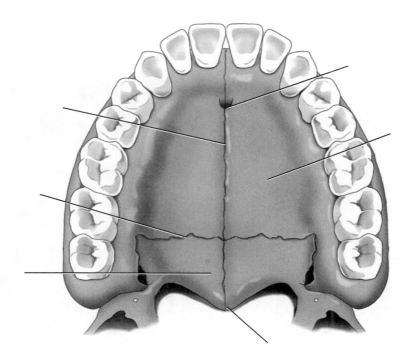

11.

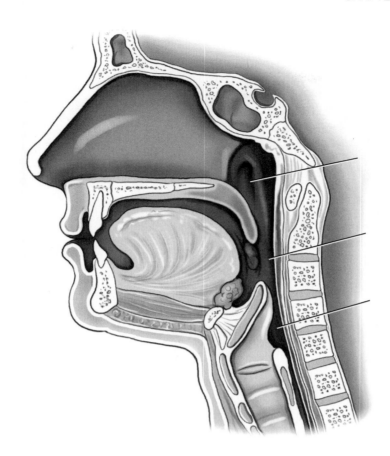

12.

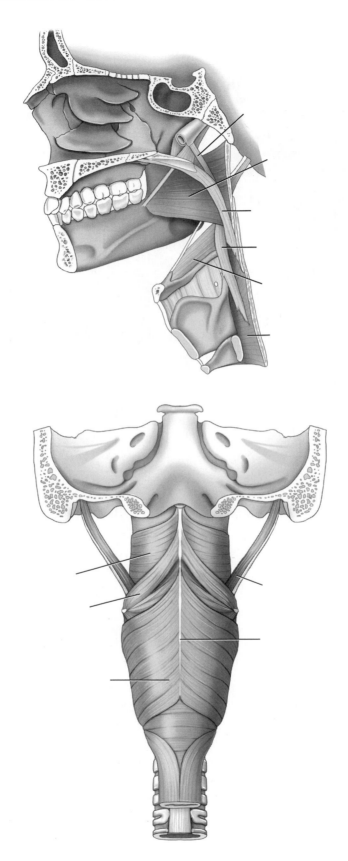

13.

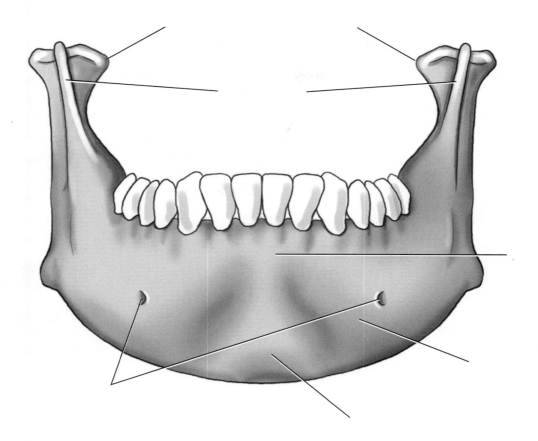

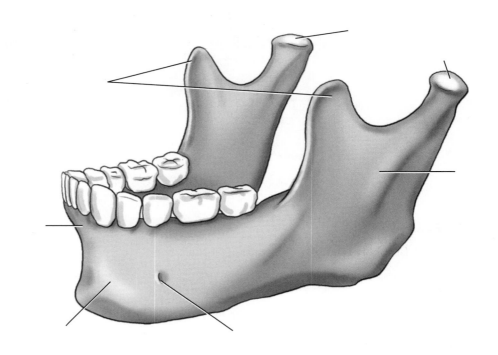

14.

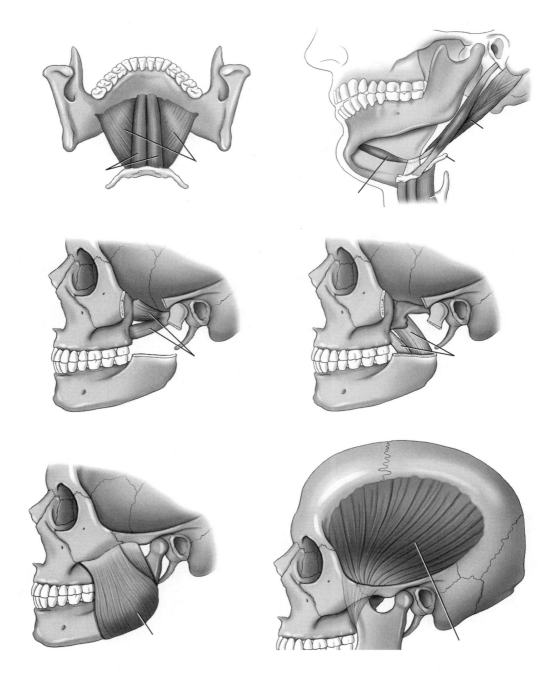

TRUE-FALSE

1. There are 8 facial bones and 14 cranial bones of the skull.

2. The articulators include the lips, tongue, teeth, palate, and tonsils.

3. In addition to its primary biological function in mastication, the mandible contributes to speech production by modifying the resonant characteristics of the oral cavity.

4. The mobility of the mandible is provided by the temporomandibular joint, which connects the maxillae to the temporal bone of the skull.

5. The tip of the tongue can move independently of the remainder of the tongue so that the tongue can coarticulate with itself. Therefore it is possible for simultaneous movement of different parts of the tongue to produce different speech sounds.

FILL IN THE BLANK

1. The muscles of the soft palate include the

   _____, _____, _____, _____, and _____.

2. The major muscle of the lips is the _____.

3. The _____ lies just behind the upper central incisors and serves as an important contact point for the production of tongue-tip sounds (e.g., /t/, /d/, /s/, /l/, and /n/).

4. Extrinsic muscles of the tongue include the
_____, _____, _____, and
_____.

MULTIPLE CHOICE

1. The primary articulator, which is responsible for the production of all English vowels and many consonants, is the
   a. hard palate
   b. teeth
   c. soft palate
   d. lips
   e. none of the above

2. Intrinsic muscles of the tongue include the:
   a. inferior longitudinal muscle
   b. genioglossus
   c. palatoglossus
   d. all of the above
   e. none of the above

3. The _____ connects the nasal cavity to the auditory tube of the middle ear, which equalizes atmospheric pressure with middle ear cavity pressure.
   a. larynx
   b. hard palate
   c. soft palate
   d. lips
   e. none of the above

4. The muscles responsible for pharyngeal movement include the:
   a. stylopharyngeus
   b. inferior, middle, and superior constrictor
   c. salpingopharyngeus
   d. all of the above
   e. none of the above

5. The muscles that elevate the mandible include the:
   a. medial pterygoid
   b. masseter
   c. temporalis
   d. all of the above
   e. none of the above

APPLICATION EXERCISES

1. Describe sound spectrography and palatometry, and explain how they are valuable aids in achieving more precise articulatory targets for communication-disordered persons, including hearing-impaired clients and those with a cleft palate.

2. Describe the source-filter theory of speech production and discuss its importance in understanding normal speech production as well as problems in speech production, including disorders affecting the source system and those that affect the filter system.

3. Define *coarticulation* and discuss its importance in diagnosing and treating articulatory disorders.

4. Describe the specific mechanism involved in achieving normal velopharyngeal closure and discuss specific causes of problems with the velopharyngeal mechanism.

5. Describe the specific role, if any, of each of the articulators in the speech production problems associated with specific disorders, including cerebral palsy, cleft palate, Parkinson's disease, amyotrophic lateral sclerosis, and hearing disorders.

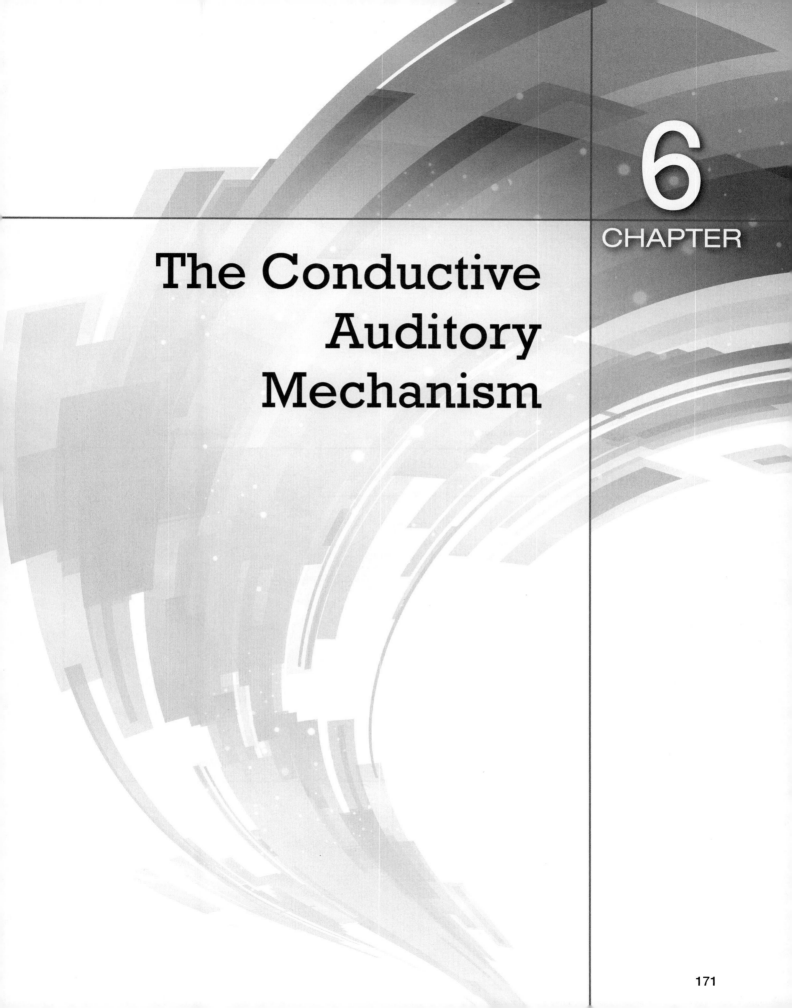

The Conductive Auditory Mechanism

The human auditory mechanism can be divided into the peripheral auditory system and the central auditory system, and subdivided still further into four divisions: outer ear, middle ear, inner ear, and central auditory system (Figure 6-1). On a functional basis, the auditory system contains three components: the conductive mechanism, the sensory mechanism, and the central mechanism. Almost all of the peripheral auditory mechanism is contained in the **temporal bone**, a paired cranial bone of the skull (Figure 6-2).

Anatomically, the conductive mechanism includes the outer ear and middle ear. Its function is to *conduct* sound energy from the outside air to the inner ear.

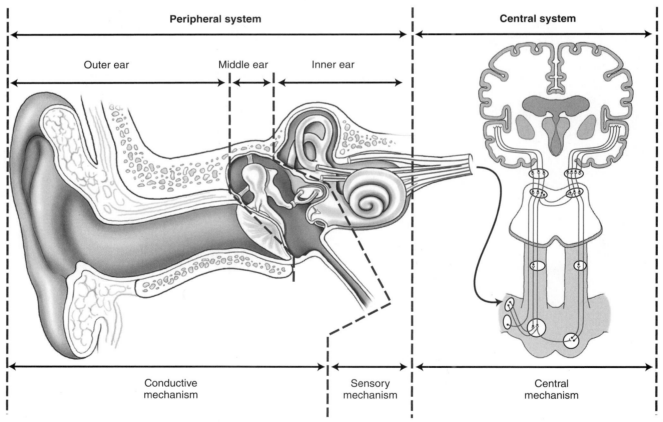

FIGURE 6-1 Human auditory mechanism.

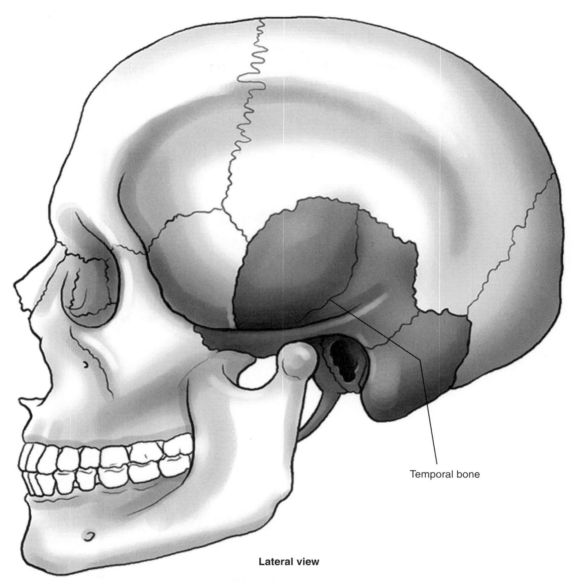

Lateral view

FIGURE 6-2 Temporal bone.

Temporal bone

OUTER EAR

The outer ear is the outermost portion of the auditory system consisting of the auricle (or pinna) and external auditory meatus (EAM). The **auricle** (Figure 6-3), the outermost portion of the conductive mechanism, is composed of soft tissue and cartilage with skin continuous with the skin of the EAM. The surface of the auricle contains ridges, grooves, pits, and depressions. In some species, like cats and dogs, the auricle may assist in collecting and directing sound energy into the EAM. However, its function is limited in humans because its muscles are vestigal and therefore of limited usefulness.

The **external auditory meatus** is a 25- to 35-mm long, very narrow (5 to 9 mm in diameter) canal that is lined with a thin layer of skin (Figure 6-4). Its lateral one-third portion is composed of cartilage, whereas its medial two thirds is bone. The cartilaginous portion of the canal is lined with hairs, which along with **cerumen** protect the tympanic membrane (eardrum) against insects and other foreign bodies. Because the EAM is S-shaped, it protects the tympanic membrane from the outside atmosphere's foreign bodies. It has two sets of glands, ceruminous (wax-secreting) and sebaceous (oil-producing).

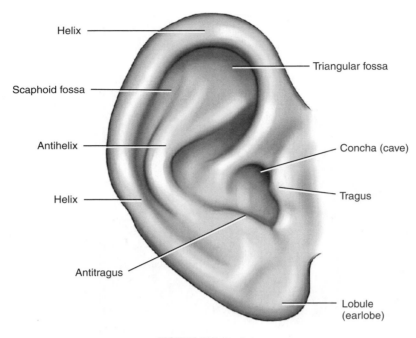

Helix

Triangular fossa

Scaphoid fossa

Antihelix

Concha (cave)

Helix

Tragus

Antitragus

Lobule
(earlobe)

FIGURE 6-3 Auricle.

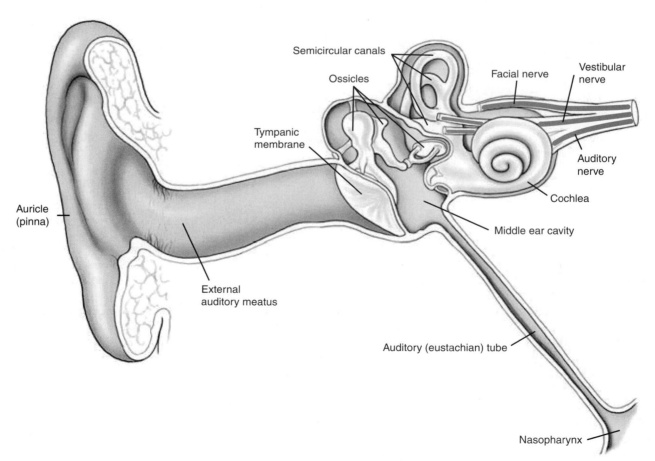

Semicircular canals

Ossicles

Facial nerve

Vestibular
nerve

Tympanic
membrane

Auditory
nerve

Cochlea

Auricle
(pinna)

Middle ear cavity

External
auditory meatus

Auditory (eustachian) tube

Nasopharynx

FIGURE 6-4 Human auditory anatomy.

TYMPANIC MEMBRANE

The **tympanic membrane (TM)** is a thin, elastic, membranous structure separating the EAM of the outer ear from the middle ear cavity (Figures 6-4 and 6-5). It varies in individuals from almost transparent to barely translucent (letting light pass through). The TM is composed of three layers of tissue: (1) an outer, **cutaneous layer** that is continuous with the lining of the EAM; (2) a middle, **fibrous layer**, responsible for the TM's compliance; and (3) an inner **mucous layer**, which is continuous with the lining of the middle ear cavity. It also has two types of fibers: (1) **radial fibers**, which begin near the center of the TM (where they are dense) and spread toward the periphery (where they are sparse); and (2) **circular fibers**, which surround the TM and are sparse near the center and dense toward the periphery.

Once the airborne acoustic signal reaches the TM, the sound is converted into mechanical vibrations of the membrane itself and remains in a mechanical mode through the middle ear.

MIDDLE EAR

The middle ear is an air-filled hollow cavity located medial to the TM (Figures 6-4 and 6-6). It is divided into the **tympanic cavity proper** (or **tympanum**) and the **epitympanic recess** (or **attic**). The tympanum comprises the majority of the middle ear cavity and includes most of the ossicular chain, and the epitympanic recess contains a small portion of the ossicular chain as well as air cells.

In the inferior, medial portion of the tympanic cavity is the orifice (internal opening) to the **auditory (eustachian) tube**, which connects the middle ear cavity to

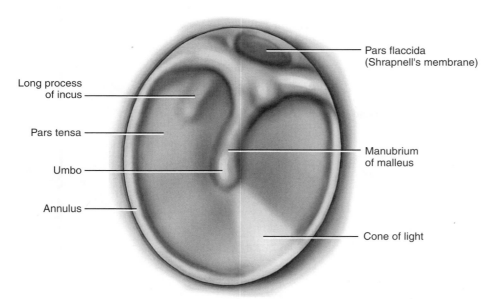

Long process of incus

Pars tensa

Umbo

Annulus

Pars flaccida (Shrapnell's membrane)

Manubrium of malleus

Cone of light

FIGURE 6-5 Tympanic membrane.

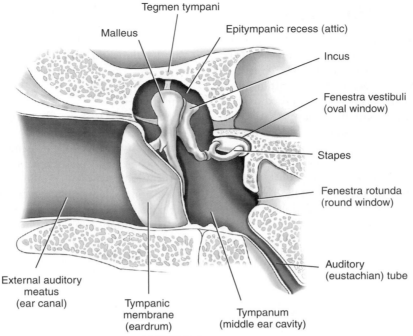

FIGURE 6-6 Middle ear.

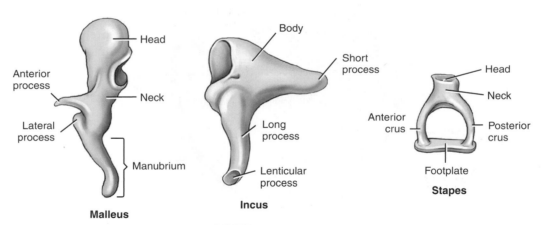

FIGURE 6-7 Ossicles.

the nasopharynx. Although usually in a closed position, the muscles of the nasopharynx open the tube during swallowing, sneezing, and yawning.

The middle ear cavity lies between the TM and the inner ear and contains air from the auditory tube. It includes three small bones (**ossicles**), the smallest in the human body, that run from its lateral to its medial walls to transmit the vibrations of the TM to the inner ear mechanism (Figures 6-6, 6-7 and 6-8). The first ossicle, the **malleus**, is attached to the TM. The second ossicle, the **incus**, is attached to the malleus via the **incudomalleolar joint**. The third ossicle, the **stapes**, is attached to the incus via the **incudostapedial joint**; its footplate is inserted into the medial wall of the middle ear cavity.

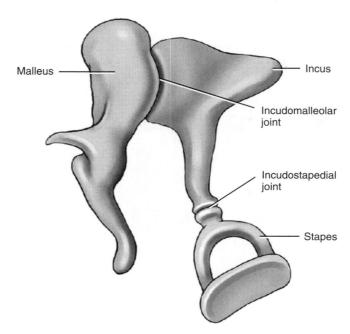

FIGURE 6-8 Ossicular chain.

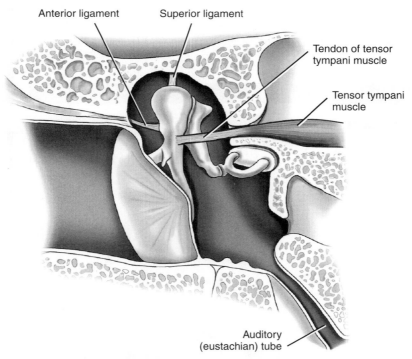

FIGURE 6-9 Ligaments of ossicular chain and tensor tympani muscle.

The ossicles are held in place by **ligaments** (Figure 6-9). Under normal conditions the ossicles vibrate in synchrony with the TM and thereby transmit the vibrations of the membrane into the inner ear.

The middle ear contains two small muscles, appropriately the smallest striated muscles in the human body because they attach to the smallest bones in the body (Figures 6-9 and 6-10). The **tensor tympani muscle** is connected via a tendon to the malleus near its neck. The **stapedius muscle** connects to the neck of the stapes via a tendon. The contraction of this muscle, which is caused by external sounds, is called the **acoustic reflex**. The most

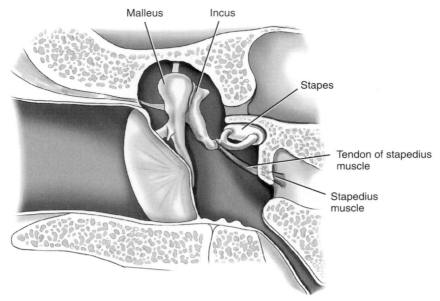

FIGURE 6-10 Stapedius muscle.

medial portion of the middle ear cavity, which separates the middle ear from the inner ear, contains two openings into the inner ear: the **fenestra vestibuli** (**oval window**) and

the smaller **fenestra rotunda** (**round window**) (Figure 6-7). Superior to the fenestra vestibuli is the **facial nerve** (**cranial nerve VII**), which passes through the middle ear (Figure 6-4).

REVIEW EXERCISES

ANATOMY EXERCISES

LEVEL 1

In the illustrations in Level 1, (a) identify each anatomical structure, and (b) identify each listed part by drawing a line to each part and labeling it.

1. _____

   helix

   scaphoid fossa

   triangular fossa

   antihelix

   concha (cave)

   tragus

   antitragus

   lobule (earlobe)

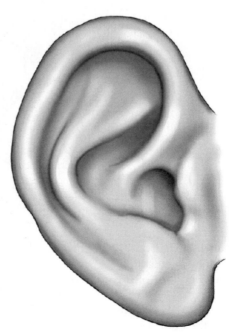

2. _____

auricle (pinna)

external auditory meatus

tympanic membrane

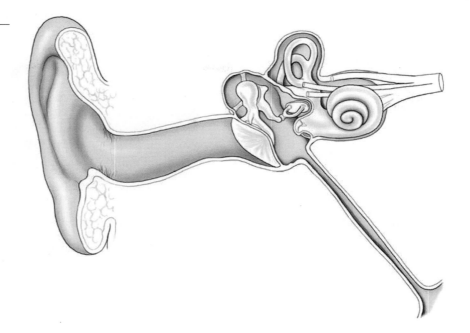

3. _____

long process of incus

pars tensa

umbo

annulus

pars flaccida

manubrium of malleus

cone of light

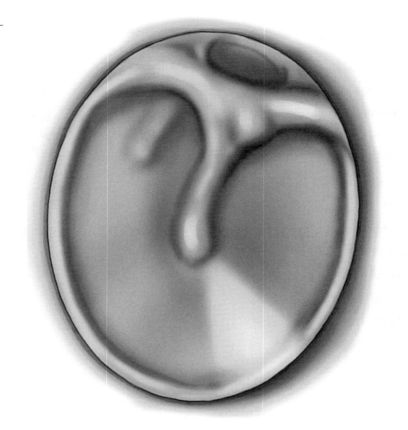

4. _____

   tympanum

   epitympanic recess

   malleus

   tegmen tympani

   incus

   fenestra vestibuli

   stapes

   fenestra rotunda

   auditory (eustachian) tube

   tympanic membrane

   external auditory meatus

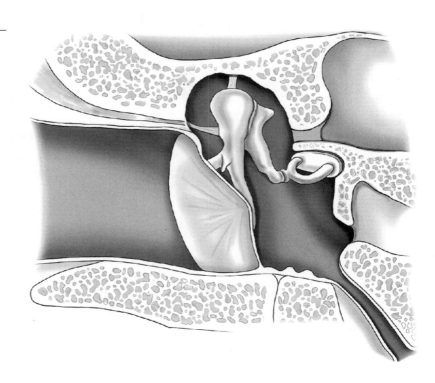

5. _____

   anterior process of malleus

   lateral process of malleus

   head of malleus

   neck of malleus

   manubrium of malleus

   body of incus

   short process of incus

   long process of incus

   lenticular process of incus

   head of stapes

   anterior crus of stapes

   neck of stapes

   posterior crus of stapes

   footplate of stapes

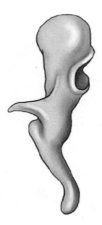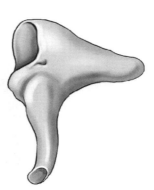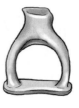

6. _____

malleus

incus

incudomalleolar joint

incudostapedial joint

stapes

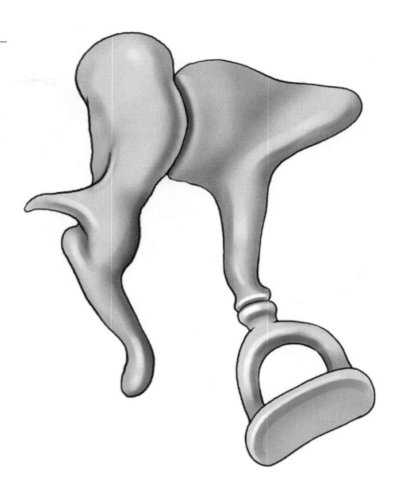

7. _____

anterior ligament

superior ligament

tendon of tensor tympani muscle

tensor tympani muscle

auditory (eustachian) tube

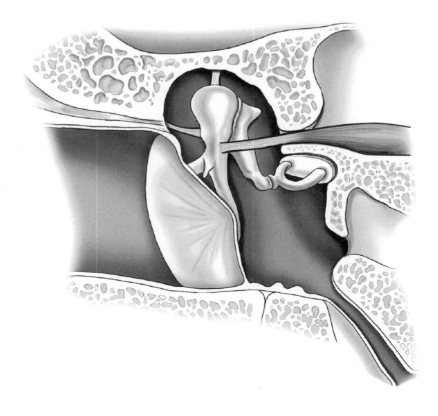

8. _____

    malleus

    incus

    stapes

    tendon of stapedius muscle

    stapedius muscle

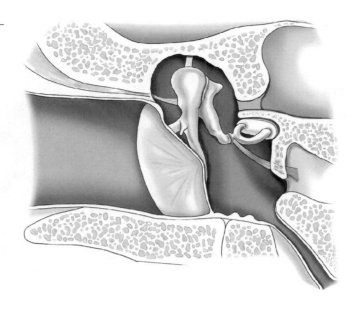

LEVEL 2

In Level 2, identify each anatomical part indicated by lines in the illustrations below.

1.

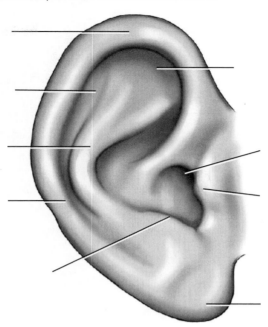

2.

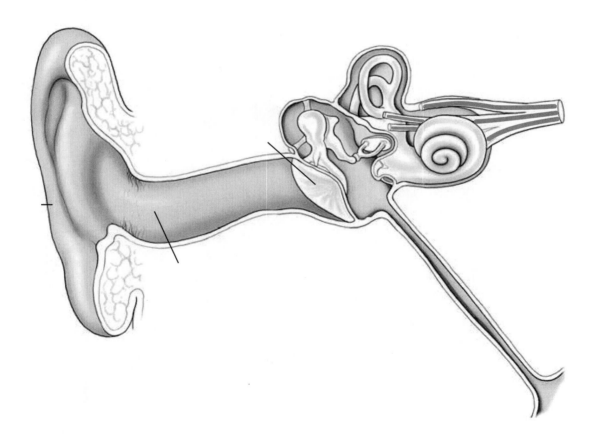

3.

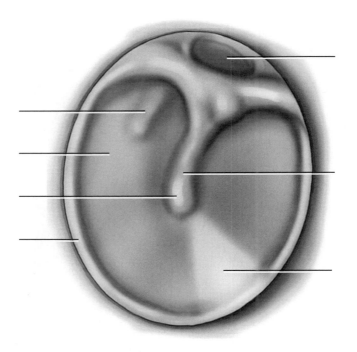

4.

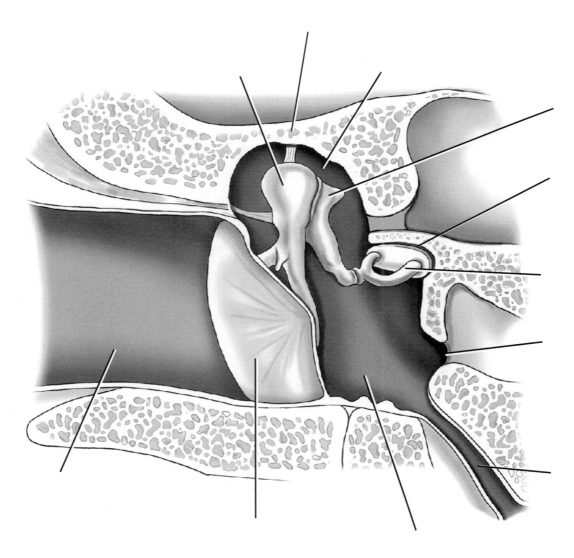

5.

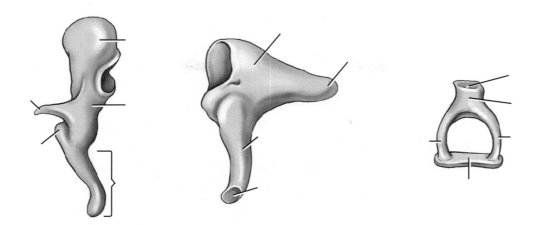

6.

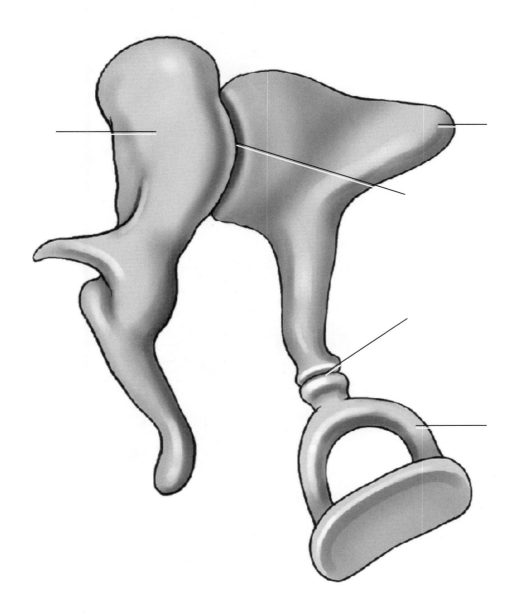

7.

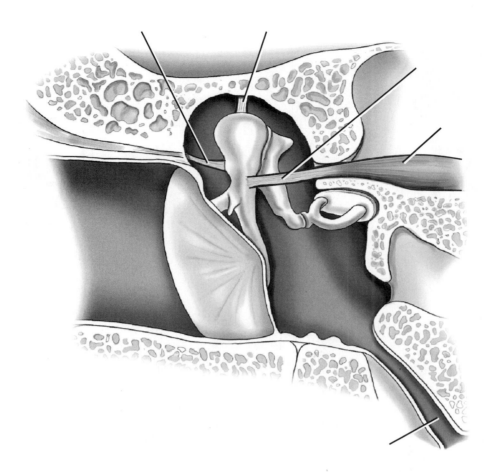

8.

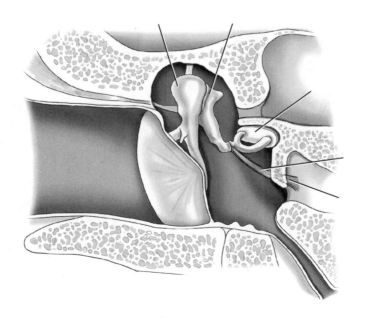

TRUE-FALSE

1. The tensor tympani muscle is attached by means of a tendon to the neck of the stapes.

2. The lateral one third of the external auditory meatus is cartilage, and its medial two thirds is bone.

3. The tympanic membrane is divided into four quadrants: anterior superior, posterior superior, anterior inferior, and posterior inferior.

FILL IN THE BLANK

1. The most lateral of the three ossicles of the middle ear is the _____.

2. The portion of the tympanic membrane containing numerous fibers that contribute to the membrane's taut nature is the _____.

3. The three ossicles that compose the ossicular chain in the middle ear are the _____, _____, and _____.

4. On a functional basis, the auditory system is composed of the _____, _____, and _____ mechanisms.

5. The two openings on the medial wall of the middle ear cavity are the _____ and _____.

6. The middle ear is divided into two anatomical areas: the _____ and the _____.

MULTIPLE CHOICE

1. A depression on the auricle that lies between the helix and antihelix is the:
   a. lobule
   b. scaphoid fossa
   c. tragus
   d. helix
   e. none of the above

2. The stapedius muscle is attached by means of a tendon to the _____ of the stapes.
   a. footplate
   b. anterior crus
   c. neck
   d. posterior crus
   e. none of the above

3. The center point of the tympanic membrane from which the cone of light radiates is the _____.
   a. pars flaccida
   b. tympanic sulcus
   c. pars tensa
   d. umbo
   e. none of the above

4. The rimlike ridge around most of the periphery of the auricle is the _____.
   a. antitragus
   b. triangular fossa
   c. lobule
   d. scaphoid fossa
   e. none of the above

APPLICATION EXERCISES

1. What are the clinical implications of the canal resonance effect in the external auditory meatus in regard to hearing testing and hearing aid fitting?

2. Describe the three mechanisms involved in middle ear function (the condensation effect, lever action of malleus and incus, and the curved-membrane buckling principle) that counteract the impedance mismatch between the air-filled middle ear cavity and the fluid-filled inner ear. Discuss their effect on the potential hearing loss that is associated with this mismatch.

3. Describe the clinical significance of the functioning of the auditory (eustachian) tube and the deleterious results of its dysfunction.

4. What is the practical significance of the middle ear musculature with regard to the prevention of damage to the auditory mechanism from very loud sounds?

5. Describe how the structure of the middle ear cavity allows for the transmission of sound energy to the inner ear.

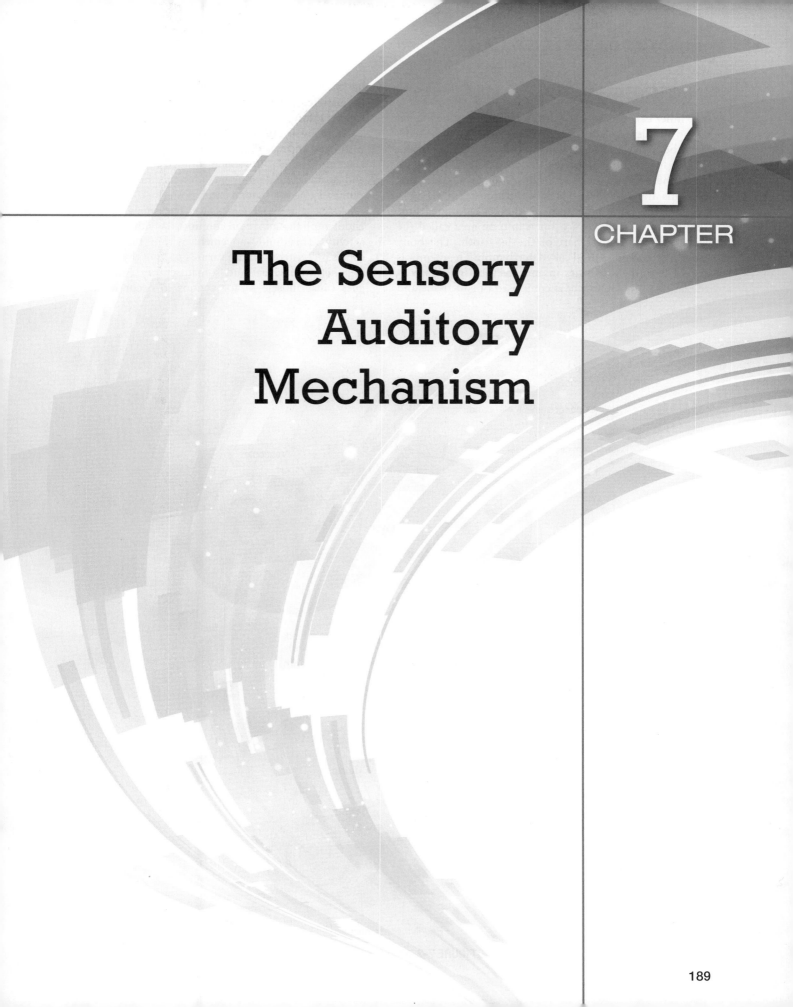

The Sensory Auditory Mechanism

7
CHAPTER

INNER EAR

The inner ear consists of fluid-filled canals that lie medial to the middle ear cavity in the petrous portion of the temporal bone. It is called the **labyrinth** because of its maze-like arrangement. The labyrinth consists of two separate parts: the **osseous (bony) labyrinth** (Figure 7-1), which contains the **membranous labyrinth** inside it (Figure 7-2). In the bony labyrinth are the **cochlea** and three **semicircular** canals, which open into an area called the **vestibule**, the central part of the labyrinth. The bony labyrinth contains a fluid called **perilymph**. The membranous labyrinth, which lies in and has the same shape as the larger bony labyrinth, is composed of soft tissue and has a series of communicating sacs and ducts, including the **utricle**, **saccule**, and **cochlear duct**. It contains a fluid called **endolymph**.

Functionally, the inner ear contains two major portions: vestibular and cochlear portions. The **vestibular portion** (Figures 7-1 and 7-2), which controls the sense of balance and spatial orientation, includes the three **semicircular canals** (superior, lateral, and posterior), each of which represents a body plane in space. The canals are filled with endolymph that moves in conjunction with head and body activity. This fluid movement within the semicircular canals is registered within various parts of the brain, which together with visual and somatosensory (muscle sense) cues cause muscle–motor actions to occur to maintain

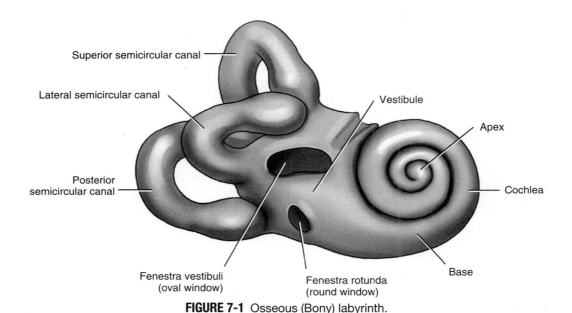

FIGURE 7-1 Osseous (Bony) labyrinth.

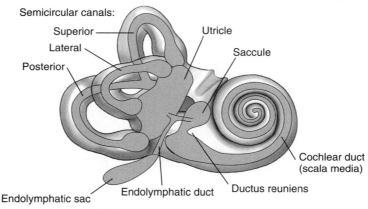

FIGURE 7-2 Membranous labyrinth.

proper body posture and stability with reference to the surrounding spatial environment.

The **cochlea** (Figure 7-1) is that part of the inner ear mechanism concerned with hearing. The inner ear communicates with the middle ear through two small windows: the **fenestra vestibuli** (**oval window**), which contains the footplate of the stapes of the ossicular chain, and the **fenestra rotunda** (**round window**), which is located slightly below the fenestra vestibuli and is covered with a thin flexible membrane to allow for expansion as fluid movements occur within the cochlea. The cochlea itself is a fluid-filled cavity divided into three canals that extend

its entire length from the base to the apex (Figures 7-3 and 7-4). The **scala vestibuli** is one of the canals; the middle canal is the **scala media** (also called the **cochlear duct**); and the **scala tympani** is the third canal. The canals are separated from each other by thin flexible membranous walls that allow fluid movement in one canal to influence fluid activity in the others. **Reissner's membrane** separates the scala vestibuli from the scala media, and the **basilar membrane** separates the scala media from the scala tympani. While the scala media is part of the membranous labyrinth, the scala vestibuli and scala tympani belong to the bony labyrinth.

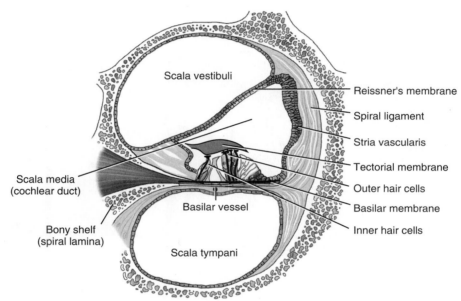

FIGURE 7-3 Scalae of the cochlea.

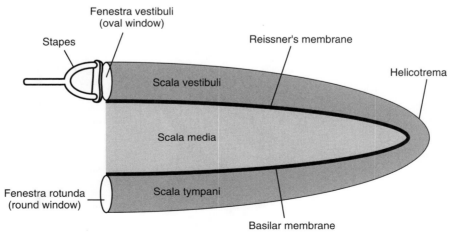

FIGURE 7-4 Schematic of the scalae of the cochlea.

The scala media contains the **organ of Corti** (Figure 7-5), the sensory end organ of hearing on the basilar membrane. It consists of approximately 3500 tiny **inner hair cells** in one row and 13,500 **outer hair cells** in three to four rows from the base to the apex of the cochlea. These hair cells serve as the sensory receptor cells for the hearing process. The **stereocilia** (or **cilia**), small hairlike projections on the tops of the inner and outer hair cells, are embedded in the **tectorial membrane** above. The basilar membrane varies in size from narrow and thin at the base of the cochlea to wider and thicker toward the apex, which results in mechanical differences related to the relative mass and stiffness of the basilar membrane.

The hair cells of the organ of Corti synapse with the nerve fibers, which group together to form the **cochlear nerve**, a branch of the eighth cranial nerve (Figure 7-6). The **vestibular nerve**, another branch of the eighth cranial nerve, originates from the semicircular canals and joins the cochlear nerve to form the **eighth cranial (statoacoustic) nerve**, sending nerve impulses from the inner ear to the brainstem and eventually to the auditory cortex of the brain.

The inner hair cells are innervated by inner fibers and the outer hair cells by outer fibers that enter the cochlea via tiny openings. These openings are collectively referred to as the **habenula perforata** (Figure 7-5). In addition to afferent innervation, both inner and outer hair cells receive efferent (descending) input.

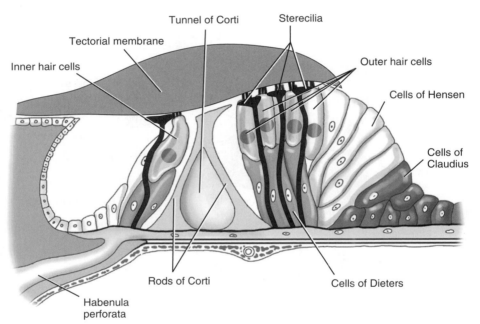

FIGURE 7-5 Organ of Corti.

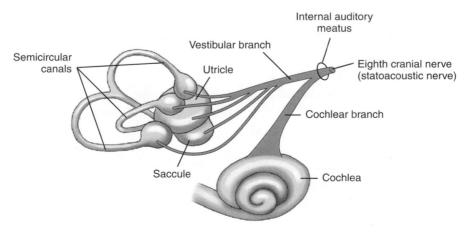

FIGURE 7-6 Cochlear and vestibular branches of the VIIIth cranial (statoacoustic) nerve.

REVIEW EXERCISES

LEVEL 1

In the illustrations in level 1, (a) identify each anatomical structure, and (b) identify each listed part by drawing a line to each part and labeling it

1. _____

superior semicircular canal

lateral semicircular canal

posterior semicircular canal

fenestra vestibuli (oval window)

fenestra rotunda (round window)

base

cochlea

apex

vestibule

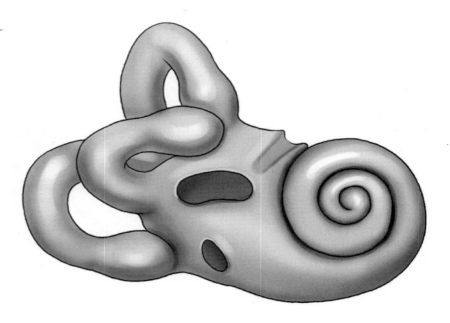

2. _____

semicircular canals: Superior

lateral

posterior

endolymphatic sac

endolymphatic duct

ductus reuniens

cochlear duct (scala media)

saccule

utricle

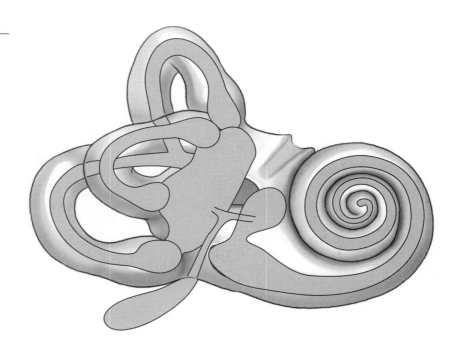

3. _____

    bony shelf (spiral lamina)

    inner hair cells

    basilar membrane

    outer hair cells

    tectorial membrane

    stria vascularis

    spiral ligament

    reissner's membrane

    scala vestibuli

    basilar vessel

    scala tympani

    scala media (cochlear duct)

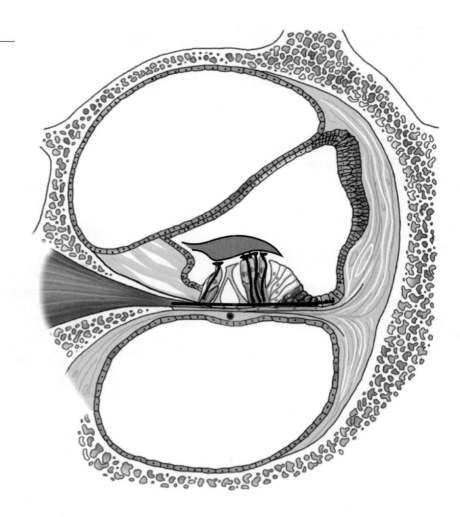

4. _____

    stapes

    fenestra rotunda (round window)

    basilar membrane

    helicotrema

    reissner's membrane

    fenestra vestibuli (oval window)

    scala vestibuli

    scala media

    scala tympani

    footplate

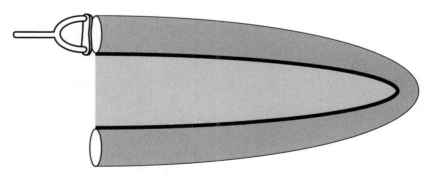

5. _____

tunnel of Corti

tectorial membrane

inner hair cells

habenula perforata

rods of Corti

cells of Dieters

cells of Claudius

cells of Hensen

outer hair cells

sterecilia

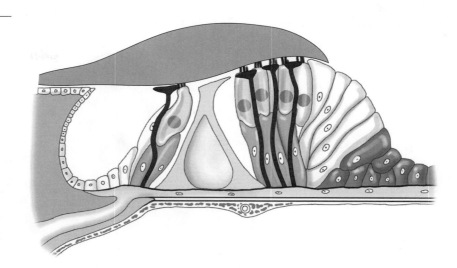

6. _____

semicircular canals

saccule

cochlea

cochlear branch

eighth cranial nerve (statoacoustic nerve)

internal auditory meatus

vestibular branch

utricle

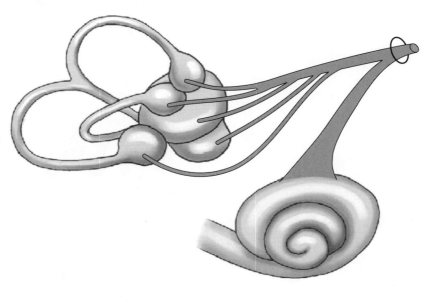

LEVEL 2

In level 2, identify each anatomical part indicated by lines in the illustrations below.

1.

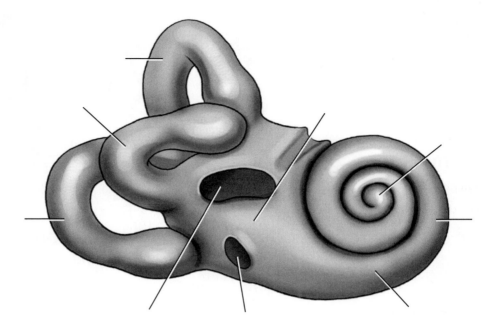

2.

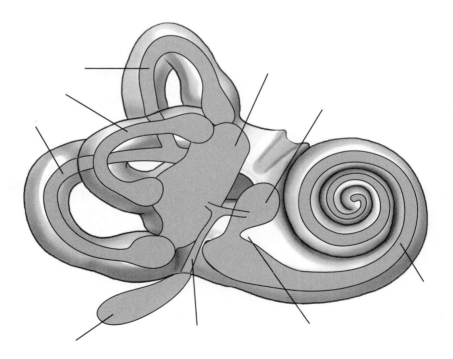

3.

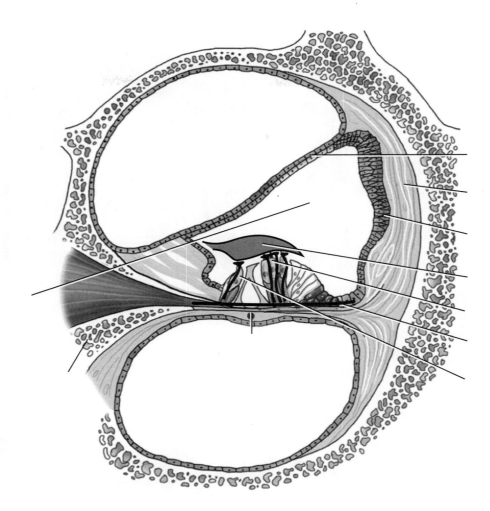

4.

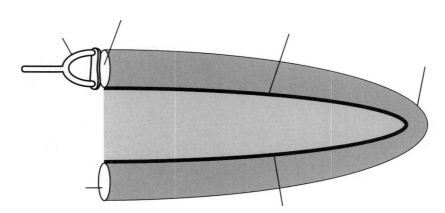

5.

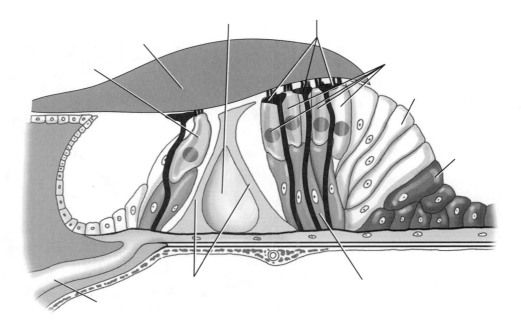

6.

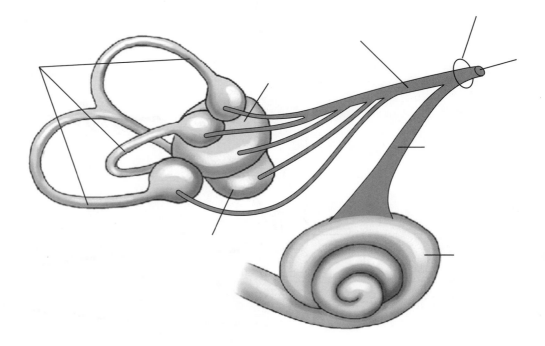

TRUE-FALSE

1. The inner ear consists of two separate parts: the membranous labyrinth and the bony labyrinth.

2. The membranous labyrinth contains a fluid called *endolymph* and the bony labyrinth has a fluid called *perilymph.*

3. The vestibular mechanism in the inner ear includes the semicircular canals and the cochlea.

4. Each of the three semicircular canals represents a body plane in space.

5. The vestibular portion of the inner ear controls the sense of balance and spatial orientation.

6. The basilar membrane is the membranous wall that separates the scala vestibuli from the scala media.

7. Whereas the scala media is part of the membranous labyrinth, the scala vestibuli and scala tympani belong to the bony labyrinth.

8. The organ of Corti is located in the scala vestibuli.

9. The hair cells in the organ of Corti serve as the sensory receptor cells for the hearing process.

FILL IN THE BLANK

1. Because of its mazelike configuration, the inner ear is referred to as the _____.

2. Functionally, the inner ear contains two major portions: the _____ portion and the _____ portion.

3. The _____ is that part of the inner ear mechanism concerned with hearing.

4. The inner ear communicates with the middle ear via two windows: the _____ and _____.

5. The cochlea is a fluid-filled cavity divided into three canals: the _____, _____, and _____.

6. The organ of Corti consists of approximately _____ inner hair cells in one row and approximately _____ outer hair cells in three to four rows.

7. The _____ nerve originates from the semicircular canals and joins the _____ nerve to form the _____ cranial nerve.

MULTIPLE CHOICE

1. The central part of the labyrinth, the area into which the cochlea and semicircular canals open, is the:
   a. cochlear duct
   b. vestibule
   c. scala media
   d. saccule
   e. none of the above

2. The inner ear communicates with the middle ear via two windows. The window that contains the footplate of the stapes is the:
   a. scala vestibuli
   b. fenestra rotunda
   c. cochlear duct
   d. scala tympani
   e. none of the above

3. The organ of Corti, the sensory end organ of hearing, is located in the
   a. scala vestibuli
   b. scala tympani
   c. scala media
   d. all of the above
   e. none of the above

4. The hair cells of the organ of Corti synapse with nerve fibers, which group together to form the _____ nerve, a branch of the eighth cranial nerve.
   a. vestibular
   b. statoacoustic
   c. cochlear
   d. labyrinth
   e. none of the above

5. The hair cells in the organ of Corti are innervated by nerve fibers that enter the cochlea by means of tiny openings collectively referred to as the:
   a. olivocochlear bundle
   b. stria vascularis
   c. superior olivary complex
   d. scala tympani
   e. none of the above

APPLICATION EXERCISES

1. Describe the mechanical, electrochemical, and active processes that contribute to the transduction (conversion) of energy that ultimately results in the detection and interpretation of the acoustic signals in our environment.

2. What are otoacoustic emissions and their clinical importance in determining the site of lesion of a hearing loss?

3. Define each of the following and describe their role in the clinical diagnosis of hearing loss:
   a. cochlear microphonic
   b. summating potential
   c. whole-nerve action potential

4. Describe the procedure for measuring the electrical activity of a single hair cell and its response to stimulation of the auditory system.

5. Define *tuning curve* and discuss its clinical significance in audiology.

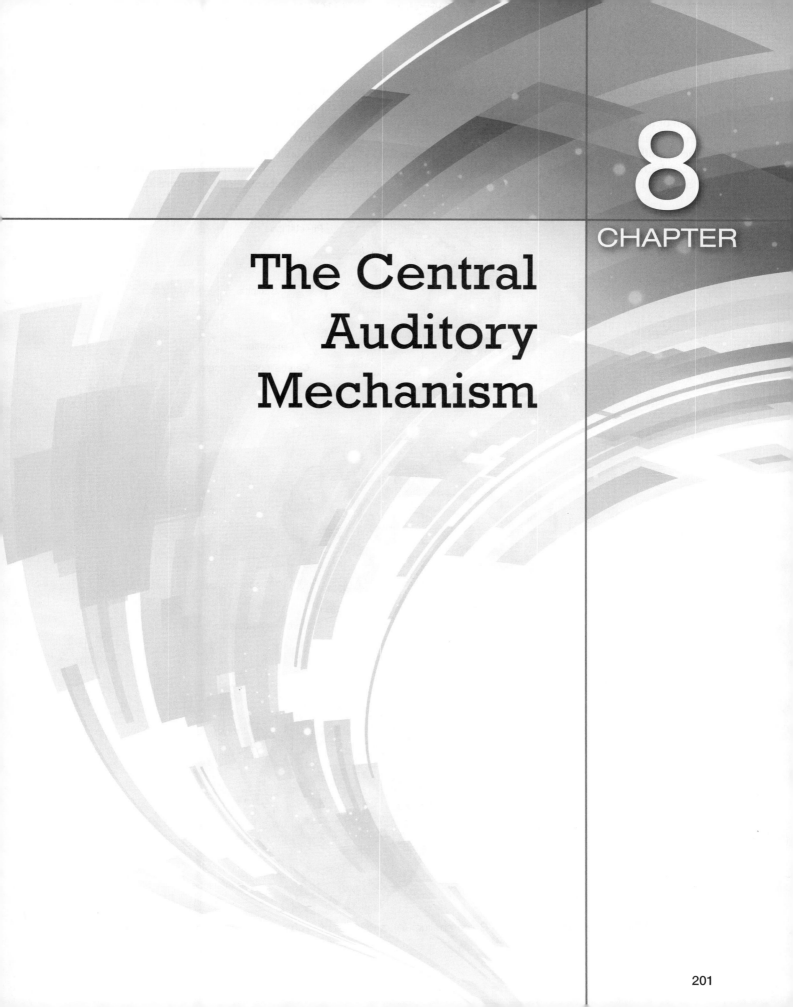

The Central Auditory Mechanism

A brief description of the overall structure of the central nervous system provides a frame of reference for the discussion of the central auditory system. The **brainstem** lies superior to the spinal cord and, in ascending order, consists of the **medulla, pons,** and **midbrain** (Figure 8-1, *A* and *B*). The **cerebellum**, the coordination center, is located just superior and posterior to the pons and midbrain. The **diencephalon** lies superior to the midbrain and contains the **thalamus** (Figure 8-1, *B*), which is a major distribution center for sensory and motor activity. Above the midbrain is the **cerebral cortex**, which is composed of two hemispheres separated by the **longitudinal fissure**. Each cerebral hemisphere contains four lobes: the **frontal, parietal, temporal,** and **occipital lobes** (Figure 8-1, *C*).

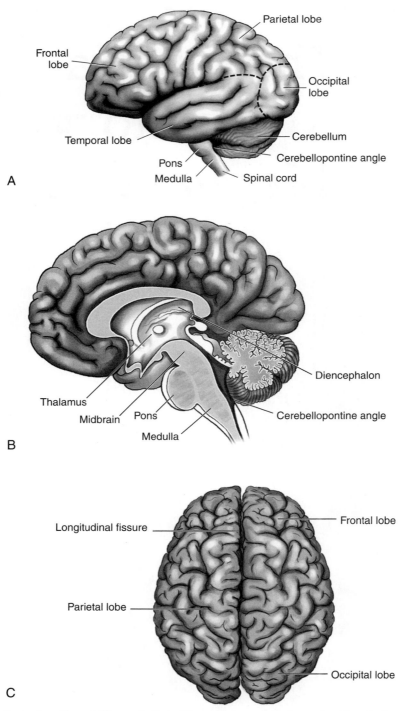

FIGURE 8-1 Brainstem (A and B), cerebellum (A), and lobes of each cerebral hemisphere (A and C).

The overall structure of the central auditory pathway is shown schematically in Figure 8-2. Upon leaving the cochlea, the eighth nerve passes through the **internal auditory meatus**, a small channel through the temporal bone that also serves as a passage for the vestibular branch of the eighth cranial (statoacoustic) nerve and the seventh cranial (facial) nerve. When leaving the internal auditory meatus, the auditory branch of the eighth nerve reaches the **cochlear nucleus**, the first major nucleus of the central auditory system. The cochlear nucleus is located at the junction of the **pons** and **medulla** in the brainstem in an area called the **cerebellopontine angle** (Figure 8-1, *A* and *B*).

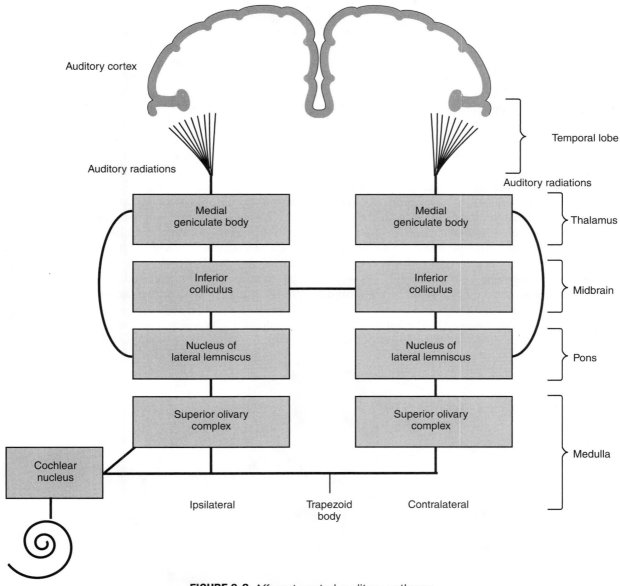

FIGURE 8-2 Afferent central auditory pathway.

AFFERENT CENTRAL AUDITORY PATHWAY

The afferent fibers of the eighth nerve terminate at the cochlear nucleus. There are two ascending pathways from the cochlear nucleus: the **ipsilateral pathway** (the pathway on the same side of the brainstem as the stimulated cochlea) and the **contralateral pathway** (the pathway on the opposite side of the brainstem as the stimulated cochlea). Approximately two thirds of nerve fibers from the cochlear nucleus cross over (**decussate**) the brainstem via a neural tract called the *trapezoid body* on the way to the next major nucleus in the medulla, the **superior olivary complex (SOC)**. The remaining one third of nerve fibers ascends to the SOC on the ipsilateral side (Figure 8-2).

The next major ascending nucleus in the pons area of the central auditory tract is the **nucleus of lateral lemniscus**, which is followed by the **inferior colliculus** in the midbrain. The two inferior colliculi are connected by fibers allowing crossover from one side of the brainstem to the other side. Some fibers from the nucleus of lateral lemniscus bypass the inferior colliculi and ascend directly to the next nucleus in the thalamus, the **medial geniculate body**. After this point, the afferent central auditory tract fans out into **auditory radiations**, multiple small fibers that connect the medial geniculate body to the **auditory cortex** in the brain's temporal lobe (Figure 8-2).

The SOC is the most peripheral point in the central auditory system to receive direct input from both cochleas, a necessity for auditory localization. The lateral nucleus of the SOC is sensitive to differences in the intensity of sound between the two ears, and the medial nucleus is sensitive to differences in the time of arrival of an auditory stimulus between the ears. This information on differences between the ears is used to localize sound. In addition, the SOC also controls the activity of both middle ear muscle reflexes (tensor tympani and stapedius). When neurological impulses from intense sounds arrive at the SOC (via the eighth cranial nerve), messages are sent down the seventh (facial) nerve to the stapedius muscle and down the fifth (trigeminal) nerve to the tensor tympani muscle, leading to contraction of the two middle ear muscles.

Much of the information from the SOC is received at the inferior colliculus either via the nucleus of lateral lemniscus or directly from the SOC. At this level, the information is synthesized and, in conjunction with visual, vestibular, and somatosensory systems, results in a localization response. In addition to localization function, the startle reflex also originates at the level of the inferior colliculus, with information relayed to the cerebellum and other higher centers.

The ascending auditory pathway proceeds to the medial geniculate body of the thalamus (Figure 8-2). The thalamus is a sensory distribution center that directs information from the sensory systems to appropriate motor and higher sensory areas of the cerebral cortex and midbrain centers (Figure 8-1, B). The medial geniculate body performs this same coordination and distribution function for auditory information. Much auditory information is directed to the **superior gyrus** of the temporal lobe (Figure 8-3) via **Heschl's gyri**. From here the information necessary for comprehension of speech is processed in **Wernicke's area** of the cerebral cortex in the posterior portion of the primary auditory area (Figure 8-3).

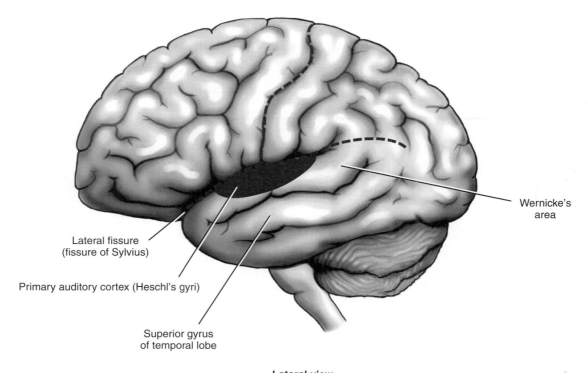

Wernicke's area

Lateral fissure (fissure of Sylvius)

Primary auditory cortex (Heschl's gyri)

Superior gyrus of temporal lobe

Lateral view

FIGURE 8-3 Primary auditory cortex.

The **auditory cortex** includes the superior gyrus of the temporal lobe and Wernicke's area on the posterior portion of the temporal lobe. It serves as the primary cortical site for processing auditory information. Moreover, it is physically larger in the left hemisphere, and there is a right-ear (left-hemisphere) advantage in processing complex acoustic signals. Based on evidence that lesions to the left hemisphere most often produce a language deficit (aphasia), the left cerebral hemisphere appears to be dominant in processing complex auditory information, including speech.

The auditory reception area is located in the temporal lobe of each of the two hemispheres of the brain. Perception of loudness and pitch and other simpler auditory behaviors are controlled at the brainstem level, while higher-level behaviors (e.g., understanding speech and the processing of other complex auditory signals) involve the auditory cortex's normal functioning. Damage to this area adversely affects the processing of complex signals, often with no effect on more basic functions (such as auditory threshold and general localization ability), which are under peripheral control.

EFFERENT CENTRAL AUDITORY PATHWAY

In addition to the afferent central auditory pathway, there is an efferent central auditory pathway of descending fibers (also called the **centrifugal pathway**), some of which originate in the brain's temporal lobe and move all the way down through the brainstem to the organ of Corti in the inner ear. The **olivocochlear bundle (OCB)**, which descends from the SOC to the organ of Corti, is an important part of this descending efferent system (Figure 8-4). It has two primary components: the **crossed olivocochlear bundle (COCB)**, which stimulates the contra-lateral cochlea, and the **uncrossed olivocochlear bundle (UOCB)**, which stimulates the ipsilateral cochlea. The COCB primarily affects inner hair cells of the contralateral cochlea, and the UOCB primarily affects outer hair cells of the ipsilateral cochlea. The effect of the activation of either COCB or UOCB is to reduce the firing rate of eighth nerve fibers that respond to a stimulus, or to worsen the threshold of those neurons for some stimuli.

The efferent auditory system is not well understood. It is known that it provides an inhibitory function, resulting in a significant increase in the intensity needed to initiate a response to an auditory stimulus thus preventing some afferent information from reaching higher centers. This inhibitory function may be related to our ability to "tune out" auditory input under certain conditions. The potential mechanical amplification provided by the outer hair cells of the cochlea may be inhibited via input through the OCB, which reduces cochlear output. Moreover, there appears to be a constant "gating" of sensory input to the cerebral cortex, with information from one sensory system having priority at one instant and another a moment later. In addition, even within the same system, it is possible to emphasize one stimulus over another, separating auditory figure from ground.

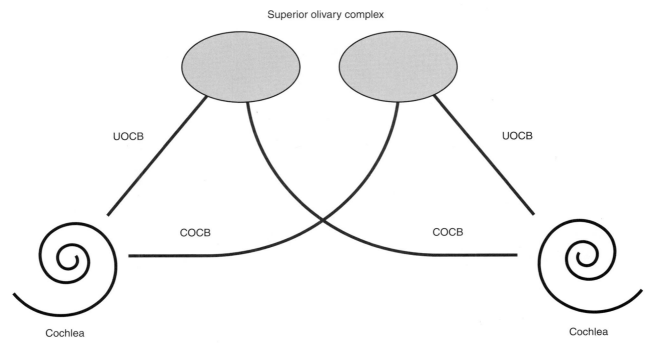

FIGURE 8-4 Efferent central auditory pathway.

SUMMARY

The central auditory system is much more than a conduit from the cochlea to the brain. The information leaving the cochlea is sorted, synthesized, and directed to appropriate portions of the central nervous system at each juncture. Moreover, actions such as the startle reflex, acoustic reflex, and localization responses are initiated at levels peripheral to the cerebral cortex, while complex analysis of speech, music, and multisensory construction of our environment take place within the cortex. Generally, function complexity increases with progression from the eighth nerve to the cerebral cortex.

In addition to the information flow from the cochlea to higher centers, there is also much neural energy flow from higher centers to lower areas, including the cochlea and the efferent system. Much of this neural activity is inhibitory or suppressive in nature. The efferent system appears to selectively limit the amount of information proceeding to the higher centers, thereby reducing "sensory overload" and allowing us to focus on sound or other sensory input that is of primary importance at a particular time.

Much can be learned about the function of the central auditory system from instances in which it is impaired, including head trauma, cerebrovascular accidents, and central auditory processing disorders, as well as through laboratory research.

REVIEW EXERCISES

LEVEL 1

In the illustrations in level 1, (a) identify each anatomical structure, and (b) identify each listed part by drawing a line to each part and labeling it.

1. A. _____

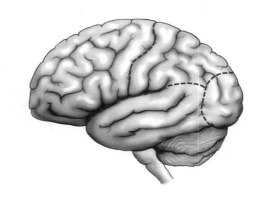

 frontal lobe

 temporal lobe

 pons

 medulla

 spinal cord

 cerebellopontine angle

 cerebellum

 occipital lobe

 parietal lobe

 B. _____

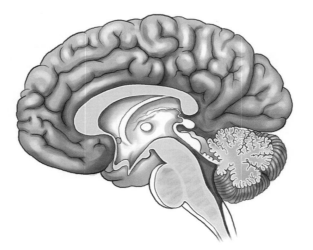

 thalamus

 pons

 medulla

 cerebellopontine angle

 diencephalon

 C. _____

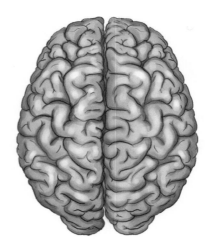

 longitudinal fissure

 parietal lobe

 occipital lobe

 frontal lobe

2. _____

auditory cortex

auditory radiations

ipsilateral

trapezoid body

contralateral

medulla

pons

midbrain

thalamus

temporal lobe

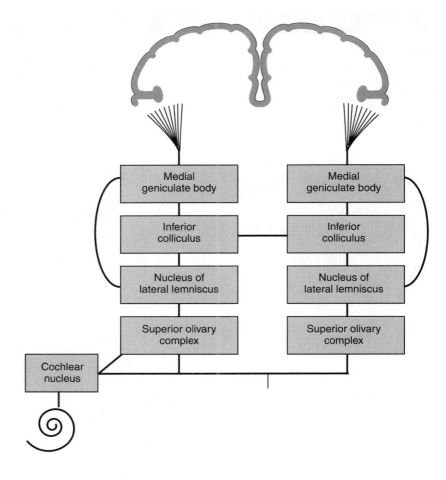

3. _____

lateral fissure (tissue of Sylvius)

primary auditory cortex (Heschl's gyri)

superior gyrus of temporal lobe

Wernicke's area

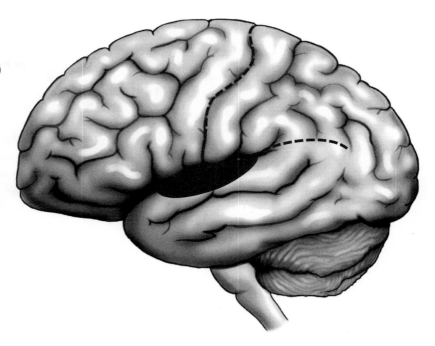

4. _____

superior olivary complex

cochlea

UOCB

COCB

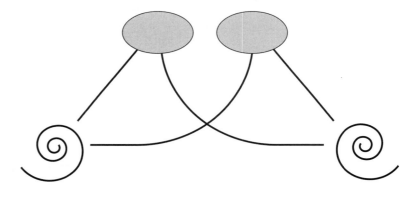

LEVEL 2
In level 2, identify each anatomical part indicated by lines in the illustrations below.

1. A.

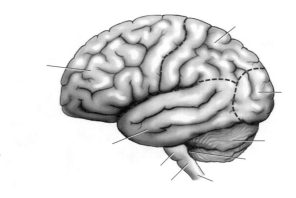

B.

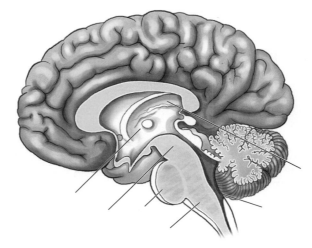

C.

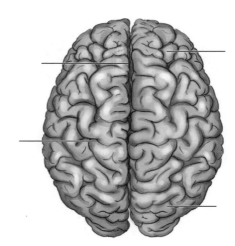

2.

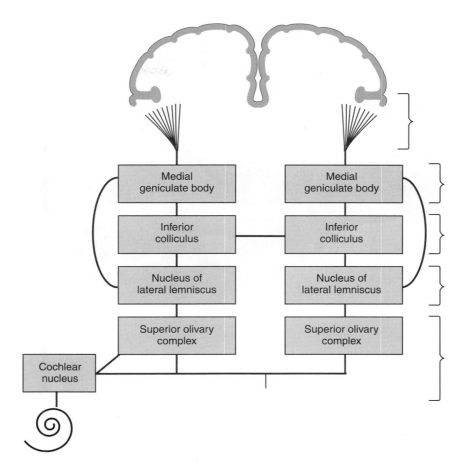

3.

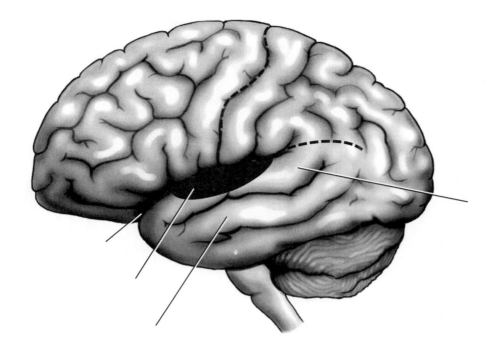

4.

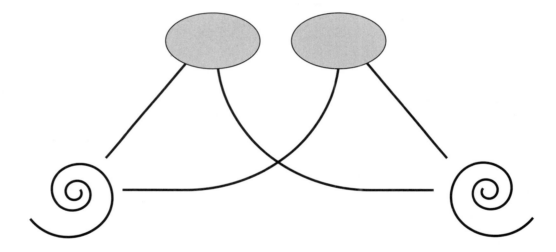

TRUE-FALSE

1. In the ascending auditory pathway, the spinal cord lies superior to the cerebellum.

2. The afferent fibers of the eighth nerve terminate at the superior olivary complex, a nucleus in the medulla that marks the beginning of the central auditory nervous system.

3. The auditory cortex is physically larger in the right than in the left hemisphere, and thus there is a right-ear advantage in processing complex auditory signals.

4. Information needed for the comprehension of speech is processed in Broca's area of the cerebral cortex.

5. The efferent central auditory system, which extends from the cerebral cortex to the cochlea, provides an inhibitory function, preventing some afferent information from reaching higher centers of the brain.

6. Actions such as the startle reflex, acoustic reflex, and localization responses are initiated at levels peripheral to the cerebral cortex, while complex analysis of speech occurs within the cortex.

7. Perception of loudness and pitch and other simpler auditory behaviors are controlled at the brainstem level.

FILL IN THE BLANK

1. Upon leaving the cochlea, the eighth nerve passes through a small channel through the temporal bone called the _____.

2. The brainstem consists of the _____, _____, and _____.

3. The _____, the coordination center, is located just superior to the pons and midbrain.

4. The _____ lies just superior to the midbrain and contains the _____, a major distribution center for sensory and motor activity.

5. Each cerebral hemisphere contains four lobes: _____, _____, _____, and _____.

6. The _____ controls the activity of both middle ear muscle reflexes (tensor tympani and stapedius).

7. The auditory cortex includes the _____ of the temporal lobe and _____ on the posterior portion of the primary auditory area.

MULTIPLE CHOICE

1. When leaving the internal auditory meatus, the auditory branch of the eighth nerve reaches the _____, the first major nucleus of the central auditory system.
   a. superior olivary complex
   b. cochlear nucleus
   c. nucleus of lateral lemniscus
   d. medial geniculate body
   e. none of the above

2. The cerebral cortex is composed of two hemispheres separated by the _____.
   a. median sulcus
   b. longitudinal fissure
   c. superior olivary complex
   d. Heschl's gyri
   e. none of the above

3. The _____ is the most peripheral point in the central auditory system to receive direct input from both cochleas, which is a requirement for auditory localization.
   a. cochlear nucleus
   b. superior olivary complex
   c. nucleus of lateral lemniscus
   d. medial geniculate body
   e. none of the above

4. The _____ is the primary cortical site for processing auditory information.
   a. auditory radiations
   b. nucleus of lateral lemniscus
   c. superior olivary complex
   d. olivocochlear bundle
   e. none of the above

5. The _____, which descends from the superior olivary complex to the organ of Corti, is an important part of the efferent central auditory pathway.
   a. superior gyrus
   b. olivocochlear bundle
   c. Heschl's gyrus
   d. inferior colliculus
   e. none of the above

6. The auditory reception area is located in the _____ lobe of each of the two hemispheres of the brain.
   a. parietal
   b. frontal
   c. temporal
   d. occipital
   e. none of the above

APPLICATION EXERCISES

1. Describe the pathway of the auditory signal from the inner ear to the brain, and discuss the implications of damage to specific portions of the central auditory pathway to the auditory process.

2. Differentiate the afferent central auditory pathway from the efferent central auditory pathway and their respective roles in the auditory process.

3. List the nuclei in the brainstem for the auditory signal on its path to the auditory cortex. Define the functional role of each nucleus in regard to audition.

4. Differentiate the function of Broca's area and Wernicke's area in the hearing process and the consequences of damage to each of these two areas.

5. Describe the interaction of the afferent and efferent central auditory pathways in normal hearing and hearing disorders.

Bibliography

Ferrand, C. T. (2007). *Speech Science: An Integrated Approach to Theory and Clinical Practice* (Second Edition). Boston: Allyn and Bacon.

Fucci, D. J., & Lass, N. J. (1999). *Fundamentals of Speech Science.* Boston: Allyn and Bacon.

Kent, R. D., & Read, C. (2002). *Acoustic Analysis of Speech* (Second Edition). San Diego: Thomson Delmar Learning.

Lass, N. J., & Woodford, C. M. (2007). *Hearing Science Fundamentals.* St. Louis & Amsterdam: Mosby-Elsevier.

Raphael, L. J., Borden, G. J., & Harris, K. S. (2011). *Speech Science Primer: Physiology, Acoustics, and Perception of Speech* (Sixth Edition). Baltimore: Lippincott Williams & Wilkins.

Schneiderman, C. R., & Potter, R. E. (2002). *Speech-Language Pathology: A Simplified Guide to Structures, Functions, and Clinical Implications.* San Diego: Academic Press.

Seikel, J. A., King, D. W., & Drumright, D. G. (2010). *Anatomy and Physiology for Speech, Language, and Hearing* (Fourth Edition). Clifton Park, NY: Delmar Cengage Learning.

Speaks, C. E. (2005). *Introduction to Sound: Acoustics for the Hearing and Speech Sciences* (Third Edition). Clifton Park, NY: Delmar Cengage Learning.

Yost, W. A. (2007). *Fundamentals of Hearing: An Introduction* (Fifth Edition). New York: Academic Press.

Zemlin, W. R. (1998). *Speech and Hearing Science: Anatomy and Physiology* (Fourth Edition). Boston: Allyn and Bacon.

Review Exercises

CHA
TR
1.
2.
3

waves. (FALSE—
s)

nplest kind of sound wave
medium. (TRUE)

mplete cycles of vibration
LSE—FREQUENCY)

a shorter period than a
E)

h the medium of air is
FALSE—340 METERS/SEC)

vibration involves first a
mpression) followed by a
nsion). (TRUE)

nitting medium increases,
und waves in that medium.
INCREASES, VELOCITY

rticles of the medium move in
ation as the wave is a trans-
LONGITUDINAL WAVE)

ound is increased, its wave-
r, and as frequency is decreased,
. (TRUE)

nds can be mathematically
r individual pure tone
in terms of frequency,
se relations with respect to one

sounds, the frequency of each
t is a whole-number multiple of
the lowest frequency. (TRUE)

ra are used to display the
litude of the component pure
complex aperiodic sounds.
EX PERIODIC SOUNDS)

odic sounds, energy is distributed
und spectrum at a particular instant

14. For a tube closed at one end and open at the other end (with uniform cross-sectional dimensions throughout its length), as tube length increases, the natural (resonant) frequencies of vibration for the tube become higher and, conversely, as tube length decreases, the natural (resonant) frequencies of vibration for the tube become lower. (FALSE—TUBE LENGTH AND RESONANT FREQUENCY ARE INVERSELY RELATED)

15. A straight tube (one that is uniform in cross-sectional dimensions throughout its length) closed at one end and open at the other end can be multiply resonant when excited by a sound source containing more than a single natural frequency of vibration. (TRUE)

16. Cavities and tubes can serve as resonators because they contain a column of air capable of vibrating at certain frequencies (their resonant or natural frequencies). (TRUE)

FILL IN THE BLANK

1. The components necessary for the creation of sound include _____, _____, and _____. (ENERGY SOURCE, BODY CAPABLE OF VIBRATION, TRANSMITTING MEDIUM)

2. The properties common to the medium of air and other media used for the transmission of sound waves are _____, _____, and _____. (MASS, ELASTICITY, INERTIA)

3. The spatial concept that refers to the maximum displacement of the particles of a medium and is related perceptually to the loudness of a sound is called _____. (AMPLITUDE)

4. _____ is the physical property of a medium that allows it to resist permanent distortion to its original shape or its molecules. (ELASTICITY)

5. _____ is the time it takes to complete one cycle of vibration. (PERIOD)

6. The velocity of sound varies as a function of the _____, _____, and _____ of the transmitting medium. (ELASTICITY, DENSITY, TEMPERATURE)

217

7. _____ is a spatial concept defined as the distance between points of identical phase in two adjacent cycles of a wave. (**WAVELENGTH**)

8. A graph that displays the frequency and amplitude of the pure tone components of a complex sound is called a _____. (**SPECTRUM**)

9. In complex periodic sounds, the pure tone component with the lowest frequency is called the _____ and the pure tone components above it that are whole-number multiples of it are called _____. (**FUNDAMENTAL, HARMONICS**)

10. _____ is the phenomenon whereby a body, which has a natural tendency to vibrate at a certain frequency (its natural or resonant frequency), can be set into vibration by another body whose frequency of vibration is identical or very similar to the resonant or natural frequency of vibration of the first body. (**RESONANCE**)

11. _____ is a graph of the frequencies to which a resonator will respond (resonate). (**FREQUENCY RESPONSE CURVE OR RESONANCE CURVE**)

MULTIPLE CHOICE

1. A physical property common to all matter that allows a body in motion to remain in motion and a body at rest to remain at rest (unless acted on by an external force) is called:
   a. elasticity
   b. impedance
   c. **INERTIA***
   d. damping
   e. none of the above

2. A time concept that refers to the movement of a vibrator from rest position to maximum displacement in one direction, back to rest position, to maximum displacement in the opposite direction, and back again to rest position, is:
   a. period
   b. frequency
   c. amplitude
   d. wavelength
   e. **NONE OF THE ABOVE* (CYCLE)**

3. The perceptual correlate of frequency of a sound is:
   a. loudness
   b. quality
   c. **PITCH***
   d. rate
   e. none of the above

4. Noise is an example of a _____ sound.
   a. simple periodic
   b. complex periodic
   c. simple aperiodic
   d. **COMPLEX APERIODIC***
   e. none of the above

COMPUTATIONAL PROBLEMS

1. The period of a 50 Hz sound traveling through air is _____ sec.
   a. 50
   b. **0.02***
   c. 1
   d. 45
   e. 25

2. The wavelength of a 5000 Hz sound traveling through air is _____ m/sec.
   a. 0.15
   b. 6.80
   c. 14.70
   d. **0.07***
   e. 0.23

3. The frequency of a sound wave traveling through the medium of air with a wavelength of 60 cm is _____ Hz.
   a. **566.67***
   b. 0.05
   c. 0.18
   d. 18.83
   e. 5.67

4. If the fundamental of a complex periodic sound is 500 Hz, the eighth harmonic of this sound is _____ Hz.
   a. 8000
   b. **4000***
   c. 1300
   d. 40,000
   e. 1000

5. For an inanimate tube closed at one end and open at the other end, of uniform cross-sectional dimensions throughout its length, the third resonant frequency is equal to the frequency of a sound wave whose wavelength is _____ times the length of the tube.
   a. 4
   b. 4/3
   c. 3
   d. **4/5***
   e. 1

6. The tenth resonant frequency of a 20-m tube closed at one end and open at the other end of uniform cross-sectional dimensions throughout its length is _____ Hz.
   a. 4.2
   b. **81.0***
   c. 8095.2
   d. 261.9
   e. 34.0

ound X is 10,000 dynes/cm² (Pa) and
und Y is 100 dynes/cm² (Pa). How
is sound X than sound Y?

bove

und A is 5000 watt/cm² and the
B is 5,000,000 watt/cm². How many
und B than sound A?

of the above* (30 dB)

of sound Z is 75 dynes /cm² (Pa). What
y in dB?

$$= \frac{75 \text{ dynes/cm}^2 (\text{Pa})}{0.0002 \text{ dynes/cm}^2 \ (\text{Pa})}$$

$$g = \frac{75 \text{ dynes/cm}^2 (\text{Pa})}{10^{-16} \text{ dynes/cm}^2 \ (\text{Pa})}$$

c. $20 \times \log = \dfrac{75 \text{ dynes/cm}^2 (\text{Pa})}{0.0002 \text{ dynes/cm}^2 \ (\text{Pa})}$ *

d. $10 \times \log = \dfrac{75 \text{ dynes/cm}^2 \ (\text{Pa})}{10^{-16} \text{ dynes/cm}^2 \ (\text{Pa})}$

e. none of the above

10. The power of sound Z is 2000 watt/cm². What is its
intensity in dB?

a. $10 \times \log = \dfrac{2000 \text{ watt/cm}^2}{0.0002 \text{ watt/cm}^2}$

b. $20 \times \log = \dfrac{2000 \text{ watt/cm}^2}{10^{-16} \text{ watt/cm}^2}$

c. $20 \times \log = \dfrac{2000 \text{ watt/cm}^2}{0.0002 \text{ watt/cm}^2}$

d. $10 \times \log = \dfrac{2000 \text{ watt/cm}^2}{10^{-16} \text{ watt/cm}^2}$ *

e. none of the above

P.O. Box 6349 .

CHAPTER 2
TRUE-FALSE

1. The vocal fundamental frequency is the pure tone with the lowest amplitude in the signal produced by the vocal folds. (**FALSE—GREATEST AMPLITUDE**)

2. The vocal tract is an air-filled tube and therefore can act as a resonator. (**TRUE**)

3. When the sound wave produced by the vocal folds is transmitted through the vocal tract, the tract will respond better to those components of the vocal fold signal that are at, or near, its natural (resonant) frequencies. (**TRUE**)

4. The human vocal tract is a multiply resonant tube. (**TRUE**)

5. Each vowel sound has its own unique set of formant frequencies. (**TRUE**)

6. For front vowels, as the cross-sectional area (radius, size) of the maximum constriction of the vocal tract increases, F_1 decreases. (**FALSE—F_1 ALSO INCREASES**)

7. In the speech production process, the generator system is responsible for producing the fundamental frequency and harmonics of the voice. (**TRUE**)

8. It is possible to alter vocal fundamental frequency without altering the characteristic quality of a vowel sound. (**TRUE**)

9. The human vocal tract is considered to be analogous to a tube open at both ends. (**FALSE—OPEN AT ONE END AND CLOSED AT THE OTHER END**)

10. Usually females have higher formant frequencies than males because they usually have shorter vocal tracts. (**TRUE**)

11. The acoustic energy in an individual speech sound is very small. (**TRUE**)

12. Speech sound quality (/i/ vs. /æ/ vs. /u/, etc.) is determined by the shape of the vocal tract which, in turn, is determined by movements of the articulators. (**TRUE**)

13. Complex sounds with different waveshapes have different perceived quality. (**TRUE**)

14. Speech sounds are not produced in isolation but rather occur in context (conversation) and thus are influenced by their neighboring sounds. (**TRUE**)

15. Partial assimilation involves a phonemic change from an allophone of one phoneme to an allophone of a different phoneme. (**FALSE—A PHONETIC CHANGE FROM ONE ALLOPHONE OF A PHONEME TO A DIFFERENT ALLOPHONE OF THE SAME PHONEME**)

16. Anticipatory assimilation is one in which an ongoing feature is continued to the next sound so that the sound is influenced by a preceding sound. (**FALSE—CARRYOVER ASSIMILATION**)

17. Coarticulation is the phenomenon of two articulators moving, one after the other in time, for different phonemes. (**FALSE—TWO ARTICULATORS MOVING AT THE SAME TIME FOR DIFFERENT PHONEMES**)

18. Speech is produced as a series of isolated, independent sounds, like beads of isolated phones put together on a string, one phone after another. (**FALSE—NOT ISOLATED, INDEPENDENT SOUNDS**)

19. In conversational speech phonemes do not exist as independent units, but rather overlap and merge into one continuously changing stream of sound. (**TRUE**)

20. Coarticulation occurs in the production of the word *top*, with the mandible moving for the vowel at the same time as the tongue is moving for the production of the linguaalveolar /t/. (**FALSE—NO COARTICULATION**)

FILL IN THE BLANK

1. The parts of the body involved in speech production include the _____, _____, _____, _____, _____, and _____. (**LUNGS, TRACHEA, PHARYNX, LARYNX, ORAL CAVITY, NASAL CAVITY**).

2. The theory proposed by Dr. Gunnar Fant to explain how sound produced by the vocal folds is modified by the acoustic properties of the vocal tract is called the _____ theory. (**ACOUSTIC THEORY OR SOURCE-FILTER THEORY**)

3. The _____ is the portion of the speech production mechanism that extends from the glottis to the lips and includes the larynx, pharynx, oral cavity, and nasal cavity. (**VOCAL TRACT**)

4. Stopping the flow of air completely but only momentarily via the blocking of the vocal tract with the tongue or lips and then suddenly releasing the air pressure built up behind this air blockage produces speech sounds classified as _____. (**PLOSIVES**)

5. The natural (resonant) frequencies of the human vocal tract are called _____. (**FORMANTS**)

6. The peaks in the spectra of vowels, which are the regions in which the frequency components are relatively high in amplitude, correspond to the _____ of the vocal tract. (**FORMANTS**)

7. The quantitative values of the formant frequencies of vowels depend on three physiologic factors: (**a. RADIUS [SIZE, CROSS-SECTIONAL AREA]) OF THE MAXIMUM CONSTRICTION; b. POSITION OF POINT OF MAXIMUM CONSTRICTION RELATIVE TO DISTANCE FROM GLOTTIS; c. LIPROUNDING)**

    a. _____

    b. _____

    c. _____

8. In the speech production process, the resonator system is responsible for determining the _____ of the vocal tract. (**FORMANTS**)

9. The perceptual correlate of vocal fundamental frequency is vocal _____. (**PITCH**)

10. The intensity of speech sounds is frequently expressed as a ratio rather than an absolute magnitude by using the _____ scale. (**DECIBEL**)

11. _____ is that characteristic of complex sounds (like those produced by the voice or musical instruments) that distinguishes one sound from another, even if the sounds have equal pitch and loudness. (**QUALITY**)

12. In "*eat* the vegetables," the normally linguaalveolar /t/ in *eat* is changed to a _____ /t/ so that the /t/ is "assimilated" to the place of articulation of /ð/ in *the* (i.e., the /t/ becomes more like /ð/ in its articulation). (**LINGUADENTAL**)

13. In the word *blank* the [n] is changed to [ŋ] in anticipation of the following [k]. This is an example of _____ assimilation. (**ANTICIPATORY**)

14. The /s/ in *taps* remains an [s], but the /s/ in *tabs* changes to [z]. This is an example of _____ assimilation. (**CARRYOVER**)

15. In the production of the word *two,* the speaker rounds the lips for [u] while the tongue is active for the production of [t]. This phenomenon is called _____. (**COARTICULATION**)

MULTIPLE CHOICE

1. The signal produced by the vocal folds can be characterized acoustically as a _____ signal.
    a. simple periodic
    b. complex aperiodic
    c. simple aperiodic
    d. **COMPLEX QUASI PERIODIC***
    e. none of the above

2. A method for making the airstream from the lungs audible involves constricting the vocal tract at some point along its length, with the airstream passing through the constriction becoming turbulent. This method is responsible for producing speech sounds classified as:
    a. plosives
    b. diphthongs
    c. vowels
    d. **FRICATIVES***
    e. none of the above

3. For front vowels, the chief cause of variation in F_1 is:
    a. **SIZE (RADIUS, CROSS-SECTIONAL AREA) OF MAXIMUM CONSTRICTION IN ORAL CAVITY***
    b. position of maximum constriction relative to its distance from the glottis
    c. liprounding
    d. all of the above
    e. none of the above

4. For back vowels, the chief cause of variation in F_1 is:
    a. size (radius, cross-sectional area) of maximum constriction in oral cavity
    b. **POSITION OF POINT OF MAXIMUM CONSTRICTION RELATIVE TO ITS DISTANCE FROM THE GLOTTIS***
    c. liprounding
    d. all of the above
    e. none of the above

5. For a tube open at one end and closed at the other end, and of uniform cross-sectional dimensions throughout it length, the lowest resonant frequency is equal to the frequency of a sound wave whose wavelength (λ) is _____ times the length of the tube.
    a. 10
    b. 2
    c. 5
    d. 20
    e. **NONE OF THE ABOVE* (4)**

6. Coupling the oral cavity to the nasal cavity results in:
    a. increased vocal fundamental frequency
    b. increased vocal amplitude
    c. increased vocal duration
    d. all of the above
    e. **NONE OF THE ABOVE***

7. The perceptual correlate of the spectrum of the voice is vocal:
    a. pitch
    b. loudness
    c. rate
    d. **QUALITY***
    e. none of the above

8. For speech comprehension purposes, the most important range of frequencies in the speech signal is _____ Hz.
    a. 20-20,000
    b. 250-8000
    c. 500-2000

d. **100-8000***
e. 10-20,000

COMPUTATIONAL PROBLEMS

1. For a tube open at one end and closed at the other end of uniform cross-sectional dimensions throughout its length, the *nth* resonant frequency is equal to the frequency of a sound wave whose wavelength (λ) is _____ times the length of the tube.
   a. 4/n-1
   b. 2/4n-1
   c. n/4-1
   d. **4/2n-1***
   e. none of the above

2. The third formant frequency of the average adult female vocal tract is _____ Hz.
   a. 12
   b. 2500
   c. **2833***
   d. 567
   e. 94

3. The tenth formant frequency of the average adult male vocal tract is _____ Hz.
   a. **9497***
   b. 500
   c. 10,767
   d. 95
   e. 567

4. If a speaker reads aloud a 300-word, 750-syllable reading passage in 2 minutes, her/his reading rate is _____ wps.
   a. 150
   b. **2.5***
   c. 0.4
   d. 6.25
   e. none of the above

5. If a speaker reads aloud a 500-word, 1000-syllable reading passage in 150 seconds, his/her reading rate is _____ wpm.
   a. **200***
   b. 3.3
   c. 6.7
   d. 150
   e. 400

6. If a speaker reads aloud a 520-word, 1000-syllable passage in 660 seconds, her/ his reading rate is _____ spm.
   a. **91***
   b. 5454
   c. 2836
   d. 47
   e. none of the above

7. Given the following information about a speaker's reading of a prose passage:
   1000 words
   1300 syllables
   speech time = 200 seconds
   intrasentence pause time = 70 seconds
   intersentence pause time = 30 seconds
   This speaker's syllables per second rate is ____**(4.3)**____ sps.
   This speaker's words per second rate is ____**(3.3)**____ wps.
   This speaker's speech-time ratio is ____**(0.67)**____.
   This speaker's pause-time ratio is ____**(0.33)**____.

APPLICATION EXERCISES

1. Describe the acoustic theory (source-filter theory) and discuss its importance in understanding the acoustics of speech production.

2. What are the clinical implications and applications associated with the fact that each different configuration of the vocal tract has its own unique set of formant frequencies?

3. Discuss the clinical implications and applications of the fact that the generator and resonator systems involved in speech production operate independently of each other.

4. Discuss the clinical applications and implications of the physiological and acoustic differences between the fundamental and formant frequencies of (a) female vs. male speakers and (b) children vs. adult speakers.

5. Discuss the clinical applications and implications of the presence of antiresonances when there is a coupling of the oral and nasal cavities.

6. Discuss the difference between *voice quality* and *vowel quality* and the clinical relevance of this difference.

7. Discuss the clinical implications and applications of the fact that in speech production and speech perception, pause time is an important component in overall speaking time.

8. Discuss the clinical importance of the contextual effects (sound influence phenomena) of assimilation and coarticulation in the diagnosis and treatment of articulation disorders.

CHAPTER 3
TRUE-FALSE

1. The respiratory tract includes the nasal and oral cavities, pharynx, larynx, trachea, bronchi, and lungs. **(TRUE)**

2. The lungs are divided into lobes, with three lobes in the left lung and two lobes in the right lung. **(FALSE—THREE LOBES IN RIGHT LUNG AND TWO IN LEFT LUNG)**

3. The ribs attach posteriorly to the corpus and transverse processes of thoracic vertebrae, and for all but two ribs anteriorly to the sternum by means of the ribs' costal cartilages. **(TRUE)**

4. The vertebrosternal ribs attach to the sternum via a common costal cartilage. **(FALSE—VERTEBROCHONDRAL RIBS)**

5. Ribs 10, 11, and 12 are called *floating ribs* because they do not attach to the sternum but instead are imbedded in the abdominal musculature. **(FALSE—RIB 10 IS A VERTEBROCHONDRAL RIB AND RIBS 11 AND 12 ARE FLOATING RIBS)**

6. The ribs vary in size, getting progressively larger from ribs 1 through 7 and then progressively smaller from ribs 8 through 12, giving the thoracic framework a barrel-like shape. **(TRUE)**

FILL IN THE BLANK

1. The ribs that attach to the sternum by means of a common costal cartilage are called _____ ribs. **(VERTEBROCHONDRAL)**

2. On the pelvis, the ligament that extends from the pubic symphysis to the iliac crest is the _____ ligament. **(INGUINAL)**

3. The coxal bone is a paired bone consisting of three lesser bones: the _____, _____, and _____. **(ILIUM, ISCHIUM, PUBIS)**

4. The pectoral girdle provides the attachment of the upper limbs to the torso (trunk) of the body. It is composed of two structures: the _____ and the _____. **(CLAVICLE, SCAPULA)**

5. The bony skeletal framework for respiration consists of the _____, _____, _____, and _____. **(VERTEBRAL COLUMN, RIB CAGE, PECTORAL GIRDLE, PELVIC GIRDLE)**

6. An unpaired segmented bone lying in the midline on the superior-anterior thoracic wall that fixes the ventral ends of the ribs' costal cartilages is the _____. **(STERNUM)**

MULTIPLE CHOICE

1. The primary muscles involved in lowering the ribs and sternum and thus participating in the exhalation phase of respiration are located in the _____ region of the body.
   a. thoracic
   b. neck
   c. back
   d. **ABDOMINAL***
   e. all of the above

2. The point on a rib where the rib changes direction, turning to curve anteriorly and then medially toward the anterior midline of the thorax, is called the:
   a. tubercle
   b. head
   c. shaft
   d. neck
   e. **NONE OF THE ABOVE* (ANGLE)**

3. The most posterior portion of the rib that attaches to the corpus of each thoracic vertebra is the:
   a. shaft
   b. neck
   c. **HEAD***
   d. angle
   e. none of the above

APPLICATION EXERCISES

1. Define and distinguish *intrapulmonary pressure* and *intrathoracic pressure* and describe their role in the speech production process.

2. Define and distinguish *tidal volume* and *vital capacity* and describe their importance in speech production.

3. Identify each of the types of speech breathing and describe their role in speech production.

4. Discuss the differences between *vegetative breathing* and *speech breathing* in regard to such measures as duration of inhalation vs. exhalation phases, force and control of air, and frequency of respiratory cycles per minute.

5. Define and distinguish between *air pressures* and *air-flow* and their role in the speech production process.

6. Identify instrumentation used to study respiratory quantities, including lung volumes, lung capacities, air pressures, and airflow.

7. Describe how the volume of air expended in speech breathing varies with the types of speech sounds produced.

8. What changes in speech breathing occur throughout the lifespan and why? What are the clinical implications of such changes for speech production purposes?

9. What speech breathing problems are associated with the following conditions? Why and how? What are the clinical implications of these speech breathing problems?
   a. Parkinson's disease
   b. cerebral palsy
   c. cervical spinal cord injury

CHAPTER 4

TRUE-FALSE

1. The process of phonation is involved in the production of all vowels, diphthongs, and consonants. (**FALSE—NOT VOICELESS CONSONANTS**)

2. Paired laryngeal cartilages include the arytenoid, epiglottis, and corniculate. (**FALSE—ARYTENOID AND CORNICULATE, NOT EPIGLOTTIS**)

3. Extrinsic laryngeal membranes connect the cartilages of the larynx to the hyoid bone above or the trachea below. (**TRUE**)

4. Extrinsic laryngeal muscles are classified anatomically as laryngeal elevators and laryngeal depressors. (**FALSE—FUNCTIONALLY**)

5. The lateral border of the vocal folds is attached to the thyroid cartilage, while the medial border of the vocal folds is free, unattached to any cartilage. (**TRUE**)

6. The opening of the glottis is widest during inhalation and narrowest during phonation. (**TRUE**)

7. Unpaired laryngeal cartilages include the thyroid, corniculate, and cricoid. (**FALSE—EPIGLOTTIS, NOT CORNICULATE**)

8. The superior division of the internal cavity of the larynx extends from the aditus laryngis to the true vocal folds. (**FALSE—FALSE FOLDS**)

9. Infrahyoid muscles of the larynx include the digastricus, mylohyoid, geniohyoid, and stylohyoid muscles. (**FALSE—THESE ARE SUPRA-HYOID MUSCLES**)

FILL IN THE BLANK

1. The space between the vocal folds when they are in an abducted position is called the _____. (**GLOTTIS**)

2. When the lateral cricoarytenoid muscle contracts, the _____ cartilages are pulled forward, thereby approximating their anterior portions in the midline, which approximates the _____ in the midline. (**ARYTENOID, VOCAL FOLDS**)

3. The free, unattached upper margin of the vocal folds is called the _____. (**VOCAL LIGAMENT**)

4. The contraction of the _____, _____, and _____ muscles is necessary to achieve approximation of the vocal folds in the appropriate adducted position to be set into vibration. (**TRANSVERSE ARYTENOID, OBLIQUE ARYTENOID, LATERAL CRICOARYTENOID**)

5. The laryngeal cartilages, located on top of the posterior quadrate lamina of the cricoid cartilage, are the _____ cartilages. (**ARYTENOID**)

6. An unpaired cartilage of the larynx that is shaped like a signet ring and forms the lower portion of the larynx is the _____ cartilage. (**CRICOID**)

7. A paired laryngeal ligament that extends from the superior cornua of the thyroid cartilage to the greater cornua of the hyoid bone is the _____ ligament. (**LATERAL THYROHYOID**)

8. The cricoid cartilage's posterior quadrate lamina contains two superior articular facets for the attachment of the _____ cartilages. (**ARYTENOID**)

9. The largest of the laryngeal cartilages that forms most of the anterior and lateral walls of the larynx is the _____ cartilage. (**THYROID**)

10. A bone in the neck region from which the larynx is somewhat suspended is the _____ bone. (**HYOID**)

11. The internal cavity of the larynx is divided into three main portions: _____, _____, and _____. (**VESTIBULE, VENTRICLE, SUBGLOTTIC REGION**)

MULTIPLE CHOICE

1. Extrinsic laryngeal membranes include the:
   a. conus elasticus
   b. thyroepiglottic ligament
   c. **LATERAL HYOTHYROID LIGAMENTS***
   d. all of the above
   e. none of the above

2. Suprahyoid muscles of the larynx include the:
   a. omohyoid
   b. thyrohyoid
   c. **STYLOHYOID***
   d. all of the above
   e. none of the above

3. The middle division of the internal cavity of the larynx, which extends from the false folds to the true vocal folds, is the:
   a. vestibule
   b. aditus laryngis
   c. subglottis
   d. **VENTRICLE***
   e. none of the above

4. The vocal fold adductor muscles of the larynx include the:
   a. oblique arytenoid
   b. lateral cricoarytenoid
   c. transverse arytenoid
   d. **ALL OF THE ABOVE***
   e. none of the above

5. The vocal fold tensor muscles of the larynx include the:
   a. **CRICOTHYROID***
   b. ceratocricoid
   c. thyroepiglottic
   d. all of the above
   e. none of the above

6. Extrinsic laryngeal muscle(s) of the larynx include the:
   a. lateral cricoarytenoid
   b. cricothyroid
   c. thyromuscularis
   d. all of the above
   e. **NONE OF THE ABOVE* (SUPRAHYOID AND INFRAHYOID MUSCLES)**

7. The abductor muscle(s) of the vocal folds is (are) the:
   a. lateral cricoarytenoid
   b. cricothyroid
   c. thyromuscularis
   d. all of the above
   e. **NONE OF THE ABOVE* (POSTERIOR CRICO-ARYTENOID)**

APPLICATION EXERCISES

1. Define *jitter* and *shimmer,* describe how they are measured, and discuss the clinical application of these vocal measures in the diagnosis and treatment of communication disorders.

2. Define *vocal fundamental frequency* and describe its physiological, acoustical, and perceptual determinants. What is considered the normal range of vocal fundamental frequency for children, adult females, and adult males?

3. Describe how the voice changes with age, including the effect of aging on various physiological, acoustical, and perceptual characteristics of the voice.

4. Describe vocal fold motion, including the phases of vocal fold vibration as well as the cartilaginous and muscular interactions in adduction and abduction of the vocal folds.

CHAPTER 5
TRUE-FALSE

1. There are 8 facial bones and 14 cranial bones of the skull. (**FALSE—14 FACIAL AND 8 CRANIAL BONES**)

2. The articulators include the lips, tongue, teeth, palate, and tonsils. (**FALSE—NOT TONSILS**)

3. In addition to its primary biological function in mastication, the mandible contributes to speech production by modifying the resonant characteristics of the oral cavity. (**TRUE**)

4. The mobility of the mandible is provided by the temporomandibular joint, which connects the maxillae to the temporal bone of the skull. (**FALSE—MANDIBLE, NOT MAXILLAE**)

5. The tip of the tongue can move independently of the remainder of the tongue so that the tongue can coarticulate with itself. Therefore it is possible for simultaneous movement of different parts of the tongue to produce different speech sounds. (**TRUE**)

FILL IN THE BLANK

1. The muscles of the soft palate include the _____, _____, _____, _____, and _____. (**GLOSSOPALA-TINUS, MUSCULUS UVULAE, LEVATOR VELI PALATINI, TENSOR VELI PALATINI, PHARYNGO-PALATINUS**)

2. The major muscle of the lips is the _____. (**ORBICULARIS ORIS**)

3. The _____ lies just behind the upper central incisors and serves as an important contact point for the production of tongue-tip sounds (e.g., /t/, /d/, /s/, /l/, and /n/). (**ALVEOLAR RIDGE**)

4. Extrinsic muscles of the tongue include the _____, _____, _____, and _____. (**GENIOGLOSSUS, STYLOGLOSSUS, PALATOGLOSSUS, HYOGLOSSUS**)

MULTIPLE CHOICE

1. The primary articulator, which is responsible for the production of all English vowels and many consonants, is the
   a. hard palate
   b. teeth
   c. soft palate
   d. lips
   e. **NONE OF THE ABOVE* (TONGUE)**

2. Intrinsic muscles of the tongue include the:
   a. **INFERIOR LONGITUDINAL MUSCLE***
   b. genioglossus
   c. palatoglossus
   d. all of the above
   e. none of the above

3. The _____ connects the nasal cavity to the auditory tube of the middle ear, which equalizes atmospheric pressure with middle ear cavity pressure.
   a. larynx
   b. hard palate
   c. soft palate
   d. lips
   e. **NONE OF THE ABOVE* (PHARYNX)**

4. The muscles responsible for pharyngeal movement include the:
   a. stylopharyngeus
   b. inferior, middle, and superior constrictor
   c. salpingopharyngeus
   d. **ALL OF THE ABOVE***
   e. none of the above

5. The muscles that elevate the mandible include the:
   a. medial pterygoid
   b. masseter
   c. temporalis
   d. **ALL OF THE ABOVE***
   e. none of the above

APPLICATION EXERCISES

1. Describe sound spectrography and palatometry, and explain how they are valuable aids in achieving more precise articulatory targets for communication-disordered persons, including hearing-impaired clients and those with a cleft palate.

2. Describe the source-filter theory of speech production and discuss its importance in understanding normal speech production as well as problems in speech production, including disorders affecting the source system and those that affect the filter system.

3. Define *coarticulation* and discuss its importance in diagnosing and treating articulatory disorders.

4. Describe the specific mechanism involved in achieving normal velopharyngeal closure and discuss specific causes of problems with the velopharyngeal mechanism.

5. Describe the specific role, if any, of each of the articulators in the speech production problems associated with different specific disorders, including cerebral palsy, cleft palate, Parkinson's disease, amyotrophic lateral sclerosis, and hearing disorders.

CHAPTER 6

TRUE-FALSE

1. The tensor tympani muscle is attached by means of a tendon to the neck of the stapes. (**FALSE—STAPEDIUS MUSCLE**)

2. The lateral one third of the external auditory meatus is cartilage and its medial two thirds is bone. (**TRUE**)

3. The tympanic membrane is divided into four quadrants: anterior superior, posterior superior, anterior inferior, and posterior inferior. (**TRUE**)

FILL IN THE BLANK

1. The most lateral of the three ossicles of the middle ear is the _____. (**MALLEUS**)

2. The portion of the tympanic membrane containing numerous fibers that contribute to the membrane's taut nature is the _____. (**PARS TENSA**)

3. The three ossicles that compose the ossicular chain in the middle ear are the _____, _____, and _____. (**MALLEUS, INCUS, STAPES**)

4. On a functional basis, the auditory system is composed of the _____, _____, and _____ mechanisms. (**CONDUCTIVE, SENSORY, CENTRAL**)

5. The two openings on the medial wall of the middle ear cavity are the _____ and _____. (**FENESTRA VESTIBULI, FENESTRA ROTUNDA**)

6. The middle ear is divided into two anatomical areas: the _____ and the _____. (**TYMPANUM [OR TYMPANIC CAVITY PROPER], EPITYMPANIC RECESS [OR ATTIC]**)

MULTIPLE CHOICE

1. A depression on the auricle that lies between the helix and antihelix is the:
   a. lobule
   b. **SCAPHOID FOSSA***
   c. tragus
   d. helix
   e. none of the above

2. The stapedius muscle is attached by means of a tendon to the _____ of the stapes.
   a. footplate
   b. anterior crus
   c. **NECK***
   d. posterior crus
   e. none of the above

3. The center point of the tympanic membrane from which the cone of light radiates is the _____.
   a. pars flaccida
   b. tympanic sulcus
   c. pars tensa
   d. **UMBO***
   e. none of the above

4. The rimlike ridge around most of the periphery of the auricle is the _____.
   a. antitragus
   b. triangular fossa
   c. lobule
   d. scaphoid fossa
   e. **NONE OF THE ABOVE* (HELIX)**

APPLICATION EXERCISES

1. What are the clinical implications of the canal resonance effect in the external auditory meatus in regard to hearing testing and hearing aid fitting?

2. Describe the three mechanisms involved in middle ear function (the condensation effect, lever action of malleus and incus, and the curved-membrane buckling principle) that counteract the impedance mismatch between the air-filled middle ear cavity and the fluid-filled inner ear. Discuss their effect on the potential hearing loss that is associated with this mismatch.

3. Describe the clinical significance of the functioning of the auditory (eustachian) tube and the deleterious results of its dysfunction.

4. What is the practical significance of the middle ear musculature with regard to the prevention of damage to the auditory mechanism from very loud sounds?

5. Describe how the structure of the middle ear cavity allows for the transmission of sound energy to the inner ear.

CHAPTER 7
TRUE-FALSE

1. The inner ear consists of two separate parts: the membranous labyrinth and the bony labyrinth. (**TRUE**)

2. The membranous labyrinth contains a fluid called *endolymph* and the bony labyrinth has a fluid called *perilymph*. (**TRUE**)

3. The vestibular mechanism in the inner ear includes the semicircular canals and the cochlea. (**FALSE—NOT THE COCHLEA**)

4. Each of the three semicircular canals represents a body plane in space. (**TRUE**)

5. The vestibular portion of the inner ear controls the sense of balance and spatial orientation. (**TRUE**)

6. The basilar membrane is the membranous wall that separates the scala vestibuli from the scala media. (**FALSE—REISSNER'S MEMBRANE**)

7. Whereas the scala media is part of the membranous labyrinth, the scala vestibuli and scala tympani belong to the bony labyrinth. (**TRUE**)

8. The organ of Corti is located in the scala vestibuli. (**FALSE—SCALA MEDIA**)

9. The hair cells in the organ of Corti serve as the sensory receptor cells for the hearing process. (**TRUE**)

FILL IN THE BLANK

1. Because of its mazelike configuration, the inner ear is referred to as the _____. (**LABYRINTH**)

2. Functionally, the inner ear contains two major portions: the _____ portion and the _____ portion. (**COCHLEAR, VESTIBULAR**)

3. The _____ is that part of the inner ear mechanism concerned with hearing. (**COCHLEA**)

4. The inner ear communicates with the middle ear via two windows: the _____ and _____. (**FENESTRA VESTIBULI, FENESTRA ROTUNDA**)

5. The cochlea is a fluid-filled cavity divided into three canals: the _____, _____, and _____. (**SCALA VESTIBULI, SCALA MEDIA, SCALA TYMPANI**)

6. The organ of Corti consists of approximately _____ inner hair cells in one row and approximately _____ outer hair cells in three to four rows. (**3500, 13,500**)

7. The _____ nerve originates from the semicircular canals and joins the _____ nerve to form the _____ cranial nerve. (**VESTIBULAR, COCHLEAR, EIGHTH OR STATOACOUSTIC**)

MULTIPLE CHOICE

1. The central part of the labyrinth, the area into which the cochlea and semicircular canals open, is the:
   a. cochlear duct
   b. **VESTIBULE***
   c. scala media
   d. saccule
   e. none of the above

2. The inner ear communicates with the middle ear via two windows. The window that contains the footplate of the stapes is the:
   a. scala vestibuli
   b. fenestra rotunda
   c. cochlear duct
   d. scala tympani
   e. **NONE OF THE ABOVE*** (**FENESTRA VESTIBULI**)

3. The organ of Corti, the sensory end organ of hearing, is located in the
   a. scala vestibuli
   b. scala tympani
   c. **SCALA MEDIA***
   d. all of the above
   e. none of the above

4. The hair cells of the organ of Corti synapse with nerve fibers, which group together to form the _____ nerve, a branch of the eighth cranial nerve.
   a. vestibular
   b. statoacoustic
   c. **COCHLEAR***
   d. labyrinth
   e. none of the above

5. The hair cells in the organ of Corti are innervated by nerve fibers that enter the cochlea by means of tiny openings collectively referred to as the:
   a. olivocochlear bundle
   b. stria vascularis
   c. superior olivary complex
   d. scala tympani
   e. **NONE OF THE ABOVE*** (**HABENULA PERFORATA**)

APPLICATION EXERCISES

1. Describe the mechanical, electrochemical, and active processes that contribute to the transduction (conversion) of energy that ultimately results in the detection and interpretation of the acoustic signals in our environment.

2. What are otoacoustic emissions and their clinical importance in determining the site of lesion of a hearing loss?

3. Define each of the following and describe their role in the clinical diagnosis of hearing loss:
   a. cochlear microphonic
   b. summating potential
   c. whole-nerve action potential

4. Describe the procedure for measuring the electrical activity of a single hair cell and its response to stimulation of the auditory system.

5. Define *tuning curve* and discuss its clinical significance in audiology.

CHAPTER 8
TRUE-FALSE

1. In the ascending auditory pathway, the spinal cord lies superior to the cerebellum. (**FALSE— BELOW THE CEREBELLUM**)

2. The afferent fibers of the eighth nerve terminate at the superior olivary complex, a nucleus in the medulla that marks the beginning of the central auditory nervous system. (**FALSE—AT COCHLEAR NUCLEUS**)

3. The auditory cortex is physically larger in the right than in the left hemisphere, and thus there is a right-ear advantage in processing complex auditory signals. (**FALSE—LEFT HEMISPHERE**)

4. Information needed for the comprehension of speech is processed in Broca's area of the cerebral cortex. (**FALSE—WERNICKE'S AREA**)

5. The efferent central auditory system, which extends from the cerebral cortex to the cochlea, provides an inhibitory function, preventing some afferent information from reaching higher centers of the brain. (**TRUE**)

6. Actions such as the startle reflex, acoustic reflex, and localization responses are initiated at levels peripheral to the cerebral cortex, while complex analysis of speech occurs within the cortex. (**TRUE**)

7. Perception of loudness, pitch, and other simpler auditory behaviors are controlled at the brainstem level. (**TRUE**)

FILL IN THE BLANK

1. Upon leaving the cochlea, the eighth nerve passes through a small channel through the temporal bone called the _____. (**INTERNAL AUDITORY MEATUS**)

2. The brainstem consists of the _____, _____, and _____. (**MEDULLA, PONS, MIDBRAIN**)

3. The _____, the coordination center, is located just superior to the pons and midbrain. (**CEREBELLUM**)

4. The _____ lies just superior to the midbrain and contains the _____, a major distribution center for sensory and motor activity. (**DIENCEPHALON, THALAMUS**)

5. Each cerebral hemisphere contains four lobes: _____, _____, _____, and _____. (**FRONTAL, PARIETAL, TEMPORAL, OCCIPITAL**)

6. The _____ controls the activity of both middle ear muscle reflexes (tensor tympani and stapedius). (**SUPERIOR OLIVARY COMPLEX**)

7. The auditory cortex includes the _____ of the temporal lobe and _____ on the posterior portion of the primary auditory area. (**SUPERIOR GYRUS, WERNICKE'S AREA**)

MULTIPLE CHOICE

1. When leaving the internal auditory meatus, the auditory branch of the eighth nerve reaches the _____, the first major nucleus of the central auditory system.
   a. superior olivary complex
   b. **COCHLEAR NUCLEUS***
   c. nucleus of lateral lemniscus
   d. medial geniculate body
   e. none of the above

2. The cerebral cortex is composed of two hemispheres separated by the _____.
   a. median sulcus
   b. **LONGITUDINAL FISSURE***
   c. superior olivary complex
   d. Heschl's gyri
   e. none of the above

3. The _____ is the most peripheral point in the central auditory system to receive direct input from both cochleas, which is a requirement for auditory localization.
   a. cochlear nucleus
   b. **SUPERIOR OLIVARY COMPLEX***
   c. nucleus of lateral lemniscus
   d. medial geniculate body
   e. none of the above

4. The _____ is the primary cortical site for processing auditory information.
   a. auditory radiations
   b. nucleus of lateral lemniscus
   c. superior olivary complex
   d. olivocochlear bundle
   e. **NONE OF THE ABOVE* (AUDITORY CORTEX)**

5. The _____, which descends from the superior olivary complex to the organ of Corti, is an important part of the efferent central auditory pathway.
   a. superior gyrus
   b. **OLIVOCOCHLEAR BUNDLE***
   c. Heschl's gyrus
   d. inferior colliculus
   e. none of the above

6. The auditory reception area is located in the _____ lobe of each of the two hemispheres of the brain.
   a. parietal
   b. frontal
   c. **TEMPORAL***
   d. occipital
   e. none of the above

APPLICATION EXERCISES

1. Describe the pathway of the auditory signal from the inner ear to the brain, and discuss the implications of damage to specific portions of the central auditory pathway to the auditory process.

2. Differentiate the afferent central auditory pathway from the efferent central auditory pathway and their respective roles in the auditory process.

3. List the nuclei in the brainstem for the auditory signal on its path to the auditory cortex. Define the functional role of each nucleus in regard to audition.

4. Differentiate the function of Broca's area and Wernicke's area in the hearing process and the consequences of damage to each of these two areas.

5. Describe the interaction of the afferent and efferent central auditory pathways in normal hearing and hearing disorders.